T0243546

DEADLY QUIET CITY

DEADLY QUIET CITY

TRUE STORIES FROM WUHAN

MURONG XUECUN

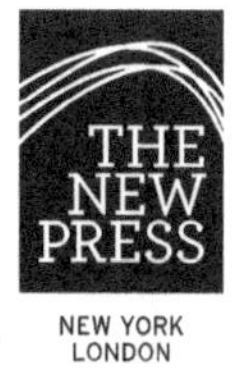

NEW YORK
LONDON

Originally published by Hardie Grant Books, Melbourne
Published in the United States by The New Press, New York, 2023
Distributed by Two Rivers Distribution

ISBN 978-1-62097-792-7 (hc)
ISBN 978-1-62097-802-3 (ebook)
CIP data is available

The New Press publishes books that promote and enrich public discussion and understanding of the issues vital to our democracy and to a more equitable world. These books are made possible by the enthusiasm of our readers; the support of a committed group of donors, large and small; the collaboration of our many partners in the independent media and the not-for-profit sector; booksellers, who often hand-sell New Press books; librarians; and above all by our authors.

www.thenewpress.com

This book was set in Sabon

Printed in the United States of America

2 4 6 8 10 9 7 5 3 1

Contents

Preface

By the time the US edition of this book arrives in the bookstores, the world will have returned to some semblance of normality. Most people will be able to walk the streets, go to work, study, and visit relatives without the constant fear of COVID-19.

The only exception will be China. A country of over 1.3 billion people will have suffered under rolling lockdowns for over three years – and the lockdowns will continue. Many people in China believe the virus is still deadly and spreading unstoppably around the world. Therefore, under no circumstances can China relax the controls. 'Even in an advanced country like America, over a million people have died,' said a friend in Beijing a few months ago. 'Look at China. How many people will die if we slack off like America?'

My friend is not uninformed or prejudiced. He is

simply making the same mistake that many Chinese people make – he believes the government. Over the past three years, the government has been incessantly repeating its narrative: 'The world is very dangerous, and you should thank us for protecting you.' Like children trapped in a cave, 1.3 billion citizens hear a wild beast howling outside the cave and they tremble in fear. Few stand up and ask what is really happening outside. If they do, in no time at all they will end up in an even darker and more confining cave.

This is in no sense benevolent, but the government is clearly benefitting a great deal. It took very little time for Xi Jinping to succeed in getting a third term. For many years to come, the Chinese people will have no choice but to submit themselves to his oppressive rule. Like leeks waiting to be harvested, as they say in China, an idiomatic phrase for suckers about to lose everything to a crooked stock manipulator.

In prosperous megacities like Shanghai, or in remote mountain hamlets, people are forced at any time into a 'state of silence,' which means no timely medical care, no leaving home to buy food, in fact no leaving home at all, like fish unable to escape the tanks at a fish monger's shop. For those who dare to break the rules, officers in full PPE will appear as soon as anyone pipes up. They will have no compunction about assaulting violators, or even tying them to a tree for public humiliation.

Many people have heard the dreaded midnight knock on the door. It means there are infections in their neighbourhood, or in their city. Just one case is enough, even an asymptomatic case, to implicate the whole neighbourhood, or the whole city. Hundreds of thousands of people have been woken by the midnight knock. Infants in swaddling and the elderly with serious illnesses are forced to leave their homes. Enduring bone-chilling winters, sweltering summers, and torrential rain, parents carry children as they support the sick and elderly, and stumble to the buses that officers allocate them to, like merchandise or livestock, destined for tightly guarded isolation centres – let's call them concentration camps.

On this vast land from Shanghai in the east to Guiyang in the southwest, hundreds of millions of Chinese people must report their location and status to the government like criminals on parole. Everyone has a personal QR code which is required to prove you are legal and uninfected just to be able to take subway journeys, enter restaurants, or shop at supermarkets. No one cares anymore about privacy or rights because they disappeared long ago in China.

In the foreseeable future, COVID-19 prevention policies that treat people with contempt will continue. When the day comes that COVID-19 is no longer a pandemic, Xi Jinping will not relinquish ruling by QR code. It will shackle China for a long time to come because the QR codes report people's movements; and when required it can be changed to ensure that 'petitioners' and dissidents, as well house church congregants, have no options to seek justice. This is an advanced technology for controlling people that even George Orwell never imagined.

Every few days, uncomplaining 'QR code citizens' line up at booths inside which there is a person, or sometimes a robot. They then squat down, open their mouths, and wait for the person, or the robot, to stick a swab down their throats or up their noses just to obtain a 'nucleic acid test visa' valid for one or two days. Only then can they legally leave their homes. But very soon they will need to apply for a new certificate, and then another and another. There will be no end to it all. If you forget to visit the testing booth, you will be reprimanded. If you try to evade testing, just wait: soon enough law enforcement officers in PPE looking like astronauts will knock on your door.

Strewn along this humiliating road lie far too many corpses. Infirm elderly have committed suicide because they cannot get medical attention; unemployed youth have leaped from buildings in desperation; unborn children have died in the wombs of mothers waiting for clearance to enter maternity wards. In the early hours of 18 September 2022, a bus full of people heading to an isolation facility crashed off the road resulting in twenty-seven deaths. Before they were taken from their homes and shoved onto that bus, they were just like us. They had dreams, unpaid debts, favourite restaurants, and loved ones ... but because they lived in China under a totalitarian rule, they were forced to leave their homes, board a bus, and die tragically at the bottom of a ravine.

Since the accident, people selected for transportation to isolation facilities are required to sign a declaration. The wording is usually abstruse, but the gist is always the same: I agree to being put into isolation and if I die, it is nothing to do with the government.

'I wonder, if I had been in the same building, how would I have avoided death,' an author posted online. 'Could I have avoided being sent to the isolation facility? Could I have avoided getting on that bus? Would I have had the courage to stand up and oppose the absurd policy?' I ask myself these questions over and over, but the answer is always, no. If I refuse to go, they will arrest me. If I stand up in opposition, they will torment my family and my children. So I have no choice other than obedience. I will obediently leave home, I will obediently get on the bus, and I will obediently hurtle to my death.

'This is my fate. But, my friends, this is not just my fate alone.'

The post disappeared in a few minutes. Perhaps the author was warned or perhaps the indefatigable censors perceived some danger and deleted the post, 'according to the law.' But the author's questions will not disappear. They await answers. How did China – once the factory of the world, the world's second largest market with countless skyscrapers and highways – come to this? What opportunities did we miss as we slid down into this abyss? Could we have rolled up our sleeves and shouted 'No!' at the dictator and saved that bus from hurtling over the cliff? And at this moment when the dictator has pushed all of China into the doomed bus, could the world do anything to save the millions of families on the bus?

*

My book does not answer these questions, but it will take the reader to the place where the disaster began, to visit the people whose voices were drowned out by the deafening noise pumped out by China's vast propaganda machine. You will hear the inner voices of people who were unable or too scared to speak out. You will share their torments. But bear in mind that these tragedies are just the beginning of an even greater tragedy.

*

On 27 July 2022, while living in Australia, I became infected with COVID-19, but unlike my compatriots I did not feel fear or concern. Instead, I felt relieved. I wrote a book about Wuhan, detailing many stories about COVID-19 but I had not actually experienced the illness myself. That had been on my conscience. 'It's all right,' I could now whisper to myself. 'I finally know what it's like.'

My symptoms were very mild, like a light cold with a slight fever and aching muscles. I recovered quickly. Australian regulations required me to isolate for a week at home and report to the government by telephone. It was a long and complicated call. The woman who answered was extremely patient as she asked me many questions. She said the government would supply free medicine and even send a nurse. Afterwards, I was in a daze for quite a while. I'm just a visitor and yet why am I treated with such care?

I lived in my socialist motherland for forty-seven years and paid plenty of taxes, but I never enjoyed any free public services. Several years ago, my then ninety-two-year-old maternal grandmother had a fall and broke her leg. She was so frugal that she constantly said, 'I'm not going for treatment. If I die, so be it.' I insisted and she reluctantly went to hospital. The operation cost 40,000 yuan [US$5,700], all of which I paid. She died in the spring of 2020 at the age of ninety-eight. Due to COVID-19 prevention policies she only had a slapdash funeral. I hope she has found peace. Now as a visitor to Australia, a country where everything is unfamiliar, I can enjoy free treatment and care. It feels like a fairy tale.

At the same time, millions of my socialist compatriots are still subject to a cruel lockdown. If a visitor from afar like me had become infected, it would quickly become a protracted nightmare. Family, neighbours, colleagues, and casual acquaintances would be dragged out of their homes and placed in isolation facilities with insufficient food. The infected person would be discriminated against and cold-shouldered for a long time. Even after being completely cured, they wouldn't be able to work or travel. The QR code that everyone must carry would remind everyone they encounter. *Look out! Here's an infected person, a dangerous and unclean infected person.*

Some observers outside of China sing the praises of Xi Jinping's Zero COVID-19 policies. They believe that although there are many problems with the policies, they have proved effective – at least in 2020, they successfully curbed the spread of the virus. I cannot agree with this view. As I see it, everything that has occurred in China over the last three years resembles the ancient parable about 'curing the hunchback.' A barbaric doctor binds a hunchback between two planks, then jumps hard on the planks. The patient's plaintive wails continue until he expires. When the family seeks out the doctor, he argues matter-of-factly: 'He came for treatment of his hunchback, and I cured his hunchback.'

*

What this book respectfully presents is those two blood-splattered planks and the plaintive wails emanating from between them. Xi Jinping's 'successes' in 2020 are not enough to eradicate those cries. And since then, the whole of China has been tied between two planks, on which Xi Jinping and his guards in white PPE are still jumping up and down.

It's time to end the praise for Xi, both within China and around the world.

The COVID-19 catastrophe delivers a sober lesson. We should not forget it was the Chinese government's deliberate coverup and misleading information that caused an epidemic in Wuhan to spread rapidly around the world. Nor should we forget that the same government's refusal to openly investigate the origins of the virus caused its provenance to become an unsolvable mystery. To this day, we do not know how it started and how it spread to humans. And we may never know.

After all this, how does the world see this dishonest and irresponsible government? When the Chinese government next ratifies a treaty or signs an agreement, will it fulfill its obligations? Are the Chinese government's promises believable? If there is another disaster like COVID-19, will the Chinese government behave honestly and responsibly? This book cannot answer these questions, but I hope it will inspire deep reflection.

*

The outbreak of the novel coronavirus began in the city of Wuhan. From space, cities look like anthills from which each day multitudes of tiny figures emerge and disperse just like busy little worker ants. The roads are crowded with little metal boxes in which they move, making a disconcerting racket. At dusk, lights come alive in an array of bright colours and stay on all night, illustrating the magnificent civilisation humankind has created. But in the spring of 2020, in a large city in the south-eastern corner of the Asian landmass, an entirely different scene appeared. The tiny creatures and little metal boxes disappeared, and all that remained was row upon row of silent structures. The once-vibrant streets were now empty and quiet.

On 23 January 2020, Xi Jinping personally ordered the city of eleven million be placed in total lockdown. All transportation links were cut, leaving millions trapped inside their own homes. During the seventy-six-day lockdown many people died silently; those who survived were tormented by fear day and night. They were anxious, frightened, and angry. They wailed plaintively for food and medicine, but hardly anyone on the outside heard them. No one knew what the millions of 'inmates' were going through and how they lived inside this catastrophe.

Herein lies the significance of this book: in the

following chapters, I will take the reader inside the city during lockdown and introduce you to the people whose voices were drowned out by the blaring official narrative. You will hear them tell their own stories.

I must admit that gathering the stories was no easy task. In China, searching for the truth can often be a criminal offence. Others went to Wuhan before me, at the most dangerous and difficult time, and we must remember their names: Fang Bin, Chen Qiushi, Li Zehua, Zhang Zhan. These citizen journalists tried everything in their quest for the truth, but all were soon arrested and silenced.

While I was in Wuhan, I often thought, 'what has happened to them could happen to me' – held in a gloomy dungeon with no sunlight, locked up alone, constantly interrogated and subjected to torture and cruel treatment, then escorted to a court to hear an imposing judge proclaim my crimes. It's a terrifying scene but not uncommon. In the past eight years, thirty-six friends of mine have been arrested. They are lawyers, journalists, and professors, all kind and honest people who have become enemies of the state simply because they have said something the government doesn't like.

I have said the same sorts of things. Before Xi Jinping came to power, I was a bestselling author. Then, because of what I wrote, all my writings were prohibited from being published and all my social media accounts were closed to my millions of followers. I became a criminal suspect, someone to be watched. The secret police would frequently come to my door. Sometimes they were polite, sometimes fierce. They forbade me from participating in certain activities and forced me to delete things I had written. Sometimes they threatened me with violence. 'You're puny,' one secret policeman said with a malevolent chuckle. 'How much beating can you take?' One freezing night not long before the novel coronavirus epidemic took hold, two policemen pounded on my door and took me to a police station. The interrogation lasted for hours, and they took detailed notes. One of them repeatedly threatened to haul me off to a detention centre. I thought I was psychologically prepared, but at that moment I discovered I would in fact tremble in fear.

You can say that this is a book about fear. I was in fear when I arrived in Wuhan, and I was in fear as I sought the truth and interviewed people. I was in fear as I wrote. Prior to publication I fled my country in fear, with all my belongings in just one suitcase. I left behind everything I had built and accumulated in my forty-seven years. I am now sitting in a coffee shop in the north of London, out of their reach, but I admit that when I recall all those times of trembling over the previous year, I still feel the heart-sinking, bitter taste of terror.

*

When the epidemic exploded, I had no thoughts of going to Wuhan. At that time, I was living in a small apartment beyond Beijing's fifth ring road. Over the course of two months, I had only gone outside three times. Like all panic-stricken Chinese people, I was frightened of being infected, though I was even more afraid of the Chinese government's epidemic prevention measures – the cutting of transportation links, the limits on movement of people, and the blocking of information. Few others were concerned about the lost freedoms and those who were dared not voice their opinions.

My neighbourhood did not have a single case of coronavirus, yet the local government still put up a fence with only one point of entry. Every time I left, I had to show the guards a small red card – my exit pass and permit to return home. Outside the fence, on the broad avenues of Beijing, there were virtually no cars or pedestrians. The traffic lights changed colour in solitude and flowers blossomed unnoticed.

I had never seen Beijing look like that before. I wondered what ground zero of the disaster might look like, 1200 kilometres away in Wuhan.

On 3 April 2020, I received a telephone call from Professor Clive Hamilton, a person I have long held in high esteem. He asked me where I was. I answered, Beijing. He sounded a little surprised. 'You're not in Wuhan?'

His question came out of the blue, but it had the effect of a sibylline enlightenment. I was momentarily stunned. I thought to myself, 'That's right. Why am I not in Wuhan?'

After Clive's phone call, I instantly saw the path forward. I knew I had to go to the locked-down city to find people who had been cut off from the world and learn about their lives to tell their stories. 'This is something you must do,' I told myself. 'Just do it, and do not think too much about the consequences.'

That afternoon, I went to a remote place on the outskirts of the city and had a long conversation with a close friend. We briefly discussed the possible dangers of the journey. My friend taught me how to set up a secure email account and how to transfer materials safely. Most importantly, my friend warned me sternly, 'Don't tell a single soul!'

I bought a train ticket, booked a hotel in Wuhan, and purchased lots of masks and sanitiser. At noon on 6 April, I quietly made my way to the train station. I kept my head down to avoid making eye contact with anyone and to evade the ubiquitous surveillance cameras. I boarded an empty train carriage like an explorer entering a dark cave, unsure what they would find.

All the way to Wuhan, no one else came into my carriage. It felt miraculous; on hundreds of trips in the past, every single train was crowded and noisy. I had never thought that a Chinese train could be so empty and so peaceful.

As I was enjoying the journey undisturbed, albeit with a sense of foreboding, my phone rang. The number was unfamiliar, and I tensed up. I have received countless calls like this and know the procedure well. I didn't answer, watching it ring until it fell silent. After a few minutes the same number called again, but this time the caller gave up impatiently after a few rings. I used another telephone to share a photograph of the screen with a friend. I commented, 'In China, we are all transparent. They know everything.'

By 'they' I meant China's secret police. I sometimes call them customer service officers. There doesn't seem to be anything they don't know. It was quite possible they had been following my movements and that my caution and care had been in vain. Perhaps they were laughing at my measures to avoid detection. By the same token, I was quite clear-eyed; a telephone call like that should not be ignored as it would provoke even more serious consequences. At the time I thought, 'Whatever is coming will arrive sooner or later; so be it.'

During my time in Wuhan, I was always on edge. I stayed at the five-star Wuhan Jin Jiang International Hotel on Xinhua Road, one of the few still open. Most of the interviews for the book were conducted in my hotel room, though on certain occasions I walked to a place by the riverbank late at night, or to a quiet street with no one else around.

Late one night, as I was going through the day's interviews, I suddenly heard voices softly talking in the corridor. Immediately, I was on my guard. I stood up, switched off the lights, and crept gingerly towards the door. I peered through the peephole looking for activity in the corridor. I saw nothing but couldn't stop feeling anxious. I frequently got up in the dark to look again at the tranquil corridor. At one moment I imagined they were about to burst through my door, which sent my heart racing. After half an hour or so I calmed down but the palms of my hands were drenched in sweat.

I was overreacting, but not without reason. Before Fang Bin disappeared, he posted a video clip on social media in which he shouted to his followers, 'They're nearby.' The young citizen journalist Li Zehua was arrested while live streaming on social media. His last words were, 'I'm being raided. I'm being raided.' Then the live stream abruptly went dead. On that chilly spring evening as I peered nervously into the darkness, I saw Fang Bin and Li Zehua. I saw their faces and their fates, and I saw myself there too.

In that same hotel room, a deeply worried Yang Min, a mother who lost her daughter, asked me, 'Is this room bugged?' I had the same misgivings. I often felt I was being followed, surveilled, and eavesdropped on; it may not have been the reality, but I couldn't prevent myself from thinking that way. All I could do was back up everything.

After each interview, the first thing I did was pass the materials on to a friend abroad. When we discussed the project, I repeatedly emphasised: 'If I am arrested, please give the materials to Clive and he will complete the book.' Publication in the West would make my life more miserable in jail, but I also knew the bad days would one day be over, no matter how wretched they might be. I thought, I'm still young enough to cope.

When friends phoned to see how I was faring, I sometimes hid under a blanket and spoke softly so as not to be snatched by the wild beast roaming about outside. I avoided talking about current affairs because it was dangerous; at most I talked about food or the weather. I would tell my friends enthusiastically, 'I'm writing a science fiction novel.' It was a lie, and a laughable one at that, but it was not entirely untrue. Some of the scenes in this book are so surreal they really do belong in a sci-fi novel.

Not everyone agreed to be interviewed. One local official said to me, 'I'm sorry, I must adhere to the regulations which prohibit interviews.' A doctor at a big hospital, whom I had telephoned several times in the hope he would talk to me, initially said he would 'think about it'. A few days later he politely turned me down.

In that interminable spring, the doctor continued to work while ill; he too was infected with the coronavirus. He must have seen bodies and perhaps shed many tears. He certainly yearned to tell someone what was on his mind but, for reasons he was afraid to reveal, he preferred to bury everything deep in his heart. 'Brother,' he said, 'I thought about it long and hard but let's just forget it. I hope you can understand it really isn't convenient.'

I said to him, 'I completely understand. I just hope that one day you will be able to tell me everything about your experience, your feelings, and what you saw and heard.'

He went silent. 'I hope so too,' he replied softly.

*

Fear is cumulative. Especially in 2020 in Wuhan. The longer I stayed, the sharper the fear became.

My hasty departure from the city was triggered by another mysterious phone call. On 4 May, a man with a Beijing accent asked me point blank, 'What are you doing in Wuhan?' I replied that I was just looking about, for no particular reason. 'Then you'd better be very careful,' the man said, sounding deeply concerned. 'You don't want to get infected because that wouldn't be good.'

To this day, I do not know what that phone call meant. Perhaps he was genuinely concerned for me, or perhaps it was another kind of warning: 'We know where you are, and we know what you're doing.'

I still had plans. I hoped to take another look at the virus laboratory; I wanted to interview many more people. At the time, Zhang Zhan was planning to help the families of coronavirus victims seek justice; I thought I could observe her and record her activities. But the mysterious phone call forced me to rethink my plans. I had already interviewed more than a dozen people and recorded more than a million words. This was my burden. The more people I interviewed, the heavier the burden became. I didn't want to risk all that.

I worked anxiously for another two days. I bought a train ticket for 7 May, travelling first to Yueyang on the opposite bank of the Yangtze River. I did not return to Beijing; with all the surveillance, it would be too risky to work on the book there. Instead, I flew to Sichuan, a mountainous province, and continued to write this dangerous book in a small town deep in the mountains.

Eight days later Zhang Zhan was arrested.

It took me ten months to write this book because there were many interruptions, the first after Zhang Zhan's arrest. The police questioned many people who had been in touch with her. A friend sent me a photo of a get-together I'd attended in early May, warning that everyone in the photograph had been questioned and that I was probably next.

I hung up the phone and stared in a daze at my draft on the computer screen. *What if something happens? What a pity it would be if I were unable to complete my task. Give me more time so I can finish it.*

There were two more mysterious phone calls, one in November 2020 and another in January 2021. Two different men called, and their tone was mild, as if they wanted to have a casual chat or send a greeting. But I was panic-stricken. After each of those calls, I put the material in a safe place, deleted everything on my computer, and waited in silence for a visitor. No one came. Perhaps the secret police were afraid of being infected.

I completed the draft in March 2021 and handed it over to my friend. The last words I wrote were: 'No matter what happens to me, this book must be published.'

My loyal friend replied: 'Understood.'

Acknowledgements

Thank you first of all to Clive Hamilton for planting the seed that has resulted in this book and for your invaluable input.

To the translator, who wishes to remain unnamed.

To Julie and the crew at Hardie Grant for your professionalism and bravery; I am deeply indebted.

To the many people who have helped me along this journey in China and around the world: you know who you are. I am truly grateful to everyone.

And finally to the people who wanted the world to know their stories: you deserve to be heard. Most appear in this book under aliases, to protect their safety.

London,
January 2022

DEADLY QUIET CITY

1.

I am a doctor, but I'm also a source of infection

Lin Qingchuan holds down a patient's tongue with a spatula and stoops over to examine his tonsils. The patient coughs reflexively. Lin feels a rush of air on his face and subconsciously pulls back.

Ten minutes later, Lin begins to feel something in his throat. 'Phlegm was constantly bubbling up like spring water,' he says later. Then the dry coughing begins. After two hours he feels weak all over, and his throat begins to ache a little, 'like a bad cold'.

He tells another doctor, 'Bad news, I hit the jackpot.'

At that time the term 'novel coronavirus' was not widely used. In a social media post to his friends, Lin says he might be infected with 'SARS plus'. A friend who is a doctor at the Wuhan No. 1 Hospital tells him,

'Don't delay. Come here right now and I'll help you get a bed.'

Lin Qingchuan declines his friend's offer. He doesn't have a fever and the symptoms are not serious, so he decides to just observe for a day. After twenty-four hours, his chest begins to hurt but he is not concerned. The next day the pain becomes acute. He has an X-ray at the radiology department of the hospital where he works, which shows the lower part of his right lung infected with the virus. He immediately contacts his friend at the Wuhan No. 1 Hospital. 'I'm really sorry,' comes the reply. 'Now even our own doctors can't get a bed.'

That was 21 January 2020. Two days later the city would be locked down, entering a seventy-six-day period of tribulation and pain. But the government's concealment of information and deception means the eleven million people of Wuhan still know next to nothing about the virus. The Lunar New Year festival is approaching, and families are busy stocking up on holiday provisions. Lin Qingchuan and his colleagues become more apprehensive by the day. They know the virus is spreading in the general population, but few people dare to speak about it publicly. 'Just protect yourself and don't blab,' Lin's family warn him.

Lin is a doctor at a small community hospital in Wuhan. Usually, he says, the hospital treats two or three cases of cold or fever each day, but in the middle of November 2019 the numbers began to rise sharply. 'In an eight-hour shift a doctor would treat twenty-five to thirty patients, of which more than half would have fevers. And many were children.'

The Chinese government is aware of the situation. It issues a type A influenza warning and orders the cessation of classes in many schools but offers no further explanation. In their social media groups, doctors begin cautiously to talk with friends, classmates and colleagues about the explosive increase in fever cases and discuss the symptoms and causes. On 8 December, someone informs Lin that the labs in the Wuhan Union Hospital or Tongji Hospital have successfully identified an atypical pneumonia virus.

From that day on, Lin Qingchuan begins to wear a face mask. Around Christmas he also dons gloves and protective goggles. Whispers of bad news multiply by the day and almost every hospital discovers infected patients. Lin tells his friends that a huge epidemic is about to break out, but few believe him. He begins to stock up on foodstuff and vegetables. Masks are still cheap – just thirteen fen, or three cents, each – and Lin buys three hundred for his elderly parents. He thinks that will be enough. 'We all thought it was an atypical pneumonia virus. No one imagined it would become such a terrible mess.'

On 31 December, the Wuhan Municipal Health Commission issues a 'situation notice' claiming that twenty-seven cases of 'viral pneumonia' have been discovered but there is no 'obvious human-to-human transmission'. It also announces that 'the disease is preventable and controllable'.

On the same day, the same organisation issues a very different internal 'emergency notification' in which the 'viral pneumonia' becomes 'pneumonia of unknown cause'. The commission requires hospitals to begin collecting infection data. Lin posts this notice on social media, adding his own comments: 'Will everybody please wear a mask, some kind of "hay typical" pneumonia is spreading.' He deliberately miswrites 'atypical' to avoid government censorship. Four hours later he adds: 'If you're smart, go and buy masks.' At dusk he posts a photo of a mask, emphasising they're essential for going outdoors.

Lin knows writing such things is a big risk. He's seen the news about eight doctors being dealt with by the police for 'spreading rumours' but feels he has an obligation to speak the truth. 'Even if only one person hears me, it would be worth it.'

On 3 January, when Hong Kong discovers its first case, Lin Qingchuan writes on social media that he hopes Hong Kong will be able to figure out what kind of pneumonia it is. He is extremely disappointed by China's 'lying government experts', whom he calls 'ex-spurts': people who 'spurt whatever their master wants them to spurt'. He asks, 'Don't your consciences hurt?'

In early January, while Wuhan is a picture of jubilation and harmony, Lin is increasingly anxious. On WeChat groups for doctors, he sees the treatment plans developed by several hospitals. But these plans do not have official endorsement. He hears news about deaths. One day in the middle of January, the entire family of a friend of Lin's is infected. They are admitted to the Wuhan Central Hospital but there are so many patients; Lin's friend tells him that there are twelve to a room and that two patients died in one night.

At this time, almost every doctor is hearing news of deaths, either by word of mouth or by witnessing them. Relatives, friends, neighbours ... so many people die and there is no way to transport the corpses in a timely manner. But in media reports and government announcements there is no mention of death, just daily exhortations to citizens not to panic: 'there are no confirmed cases of human-to-human transmission'; the disease is 'preventable and controllable'.

It isn't until 11 January that the government reluctantly announces the first death. Lin Qingchuan is incensed, and he posts a message to friends on social media: 'Raise your head three feet, god's there.' It means: 'Heaven is watching you, so beware of heaven's wrath.' A week later, he sharply criticises the government's reckless decisions: 'You send doctors to public places to check people's temperatures, but you don't supply PPE and don't permit them to wear PPE, saying you prefer us to be on high alert without showing it. What do you think we doctors are?' Nor in private does he disguise his anger. 'We know people die every day,' says Lin, 'but they continued to say: no one died, no one died. That was when we doctors lost all trust in the government.'

Recalling the situation a few months later, Lin Qingchuan's feelings are complex. Apart from anxiety and anger, he has an ineffable sense of fear. From early January one of his close friends, a doctor at the Tongji Hospital respiratory department, requested and then forced his family to take antiviral medications but didn't explain why. Only later does Lin learn that the Communist Party's feared Central Commission for Discipline Inspection and the hospital management had banned doctors from revealing the truth to the outside world. 'He was so afraid he did not even tell his wife,' Lin says of his friend. 'No one would really know if a couple whispers something, but he didn't dare to because if it were ever discovered his job and income ... everything would be over. That was the level of fear.'

*

Lin Qingchuan is not the first doctor to 'hit the jackpot', nor the last. On 21 January, eight doctors and nurses at his small hospital are infected by the virus, and in the following days the numbers grow quickly: fourteen, eighteen, twenty-two. All the frontline doctors and nurses are infected. None escape. Lin believes it would be best to close the hospital and isolate the staff. 'In the end,' he says, 'no one was left so even the accounting staff had to come in and take over.'

On 23 January, the day Wuhan is locked down, Lin has a day at home and begins self-treatment. 'A one-gram dose of amoxicillin will cure me in three to five days,' he tells his friends. He's optimistic. 'If I don't die in nine days, I won't die.'

The next day is Lunar New Year's Eve. Lin eats a simple meal: chilli peppers fried with shredded pork and a bowl of rice. He's dispirited. On social media he criticises the government harshly for failing to do its duty: 'Infected patients are not being isolated, there is no environmental disinfecting. Worse, medical personnel have not been issued PPE.' A few hours later he pleads, 'We are fighting this battle with our lungs, I'm begging you to issue us with protective goggles.'

On the evening of 25 January, Lin Qingchuan receives a notice from the hospital: all personnel must return to work. 'I'm still infectious,' he tries to reason with the hospital director. 'How can I go back to treating patients in this state?' The hospital director says he has no choice because the 'order came from upstairs. Without an official diagnosis you have to return to your post.'

His friends tell him not to go back to work, but Lin Qingchuan is thinking of his colleagues. 'If I don't go, their workload will go up. I'm a doctor, but I'm also a source of infection. What a disgrace.'

In the following days, Lin is surrounded by the chaos of the lockdown, the shortages and the incurable sorrow. In his small community hospital, there is only one box of fever medication, almost no anti-inflammatories, no protective goggles or gowns, only forty masks, and even a shortage of thermometers. Every doctor and nurse is either a 'suspected patient' or 'close contact of an infected person', but the government's strict order forces them to rush into battle, expecting to die.

Lin's condition worsens. On 28 January, while on overnight duty in the outpatient department, his chest suddenly begins to hurt. 'The kind of pain we call "end-of-life pain".' It makes him very nervous. He consults his colleagues; one doctor tells him levofloxacin might be effective because she has used it to relieve symptoms. He prescribes himself five packets of levofloxacin. The broad-spectrum antibiotics are administered by IV drip the next day and he returns to his overnight duties.

According to government regulations, the community hospital can only do triage and medical check-ups. Fever patients, regardless of how serious, have to take themselves to the Wuhan Pu'ai Hospital, a designated hospital for novel coronavirus patients. It is several kilometres from the community hospital. Because of the government ban on all vehicles during lockdown, most patients have no option but to trudge to the bigger hospital. 'Young people are strong enough to walk back but most of the old people who walk to hospital do not return.'

The Wuhan Pu'ai Hospital is a chaotic scene. Lin Qingchuan learns that at the end of January, the entire emergency department is completely 'wiped out' by the sickness. When no one can work anymore, doctors from internal medicine, orthopaedic surgery and neurology are transferred to the outpatient department. He hears that patients are flooding in and are jam-packed into every corner of the hospital. 'People were lying prone in the lobby and many couldn't even get in the front door.' Some patients ask Lin for help to get an ambulance to take them to Pu'ai. He makes many phone calls but there aren't any vehicles available. 'The emergency 120 telephone number had been overwhelmed. One day they told me there were seven hundred people in line.'

During this period, Lin Qingchuan sees countless anxious, despairing faces. He hears so much wailing and pleading, but he can offer no help because there is no medicine available and the government does not permit his hospital to treat people.

On the evening of 28 January, a woman calls Lin to say that her seventy-year-old father is losing consciousness. She implores Lin for help, but he is the only doctor on duty so cannot leave his post. A few hours later she calls again to say her father has lost consciousness, his breathing is shallow and his pulse is weak. 'Doctor, I beg you. I just need someone to help me get my father into my car so I can take him to hospital. I can't carry him to the car by myself.'

The next morning, an exhausted Lin Qingchuan leaves his hospital's outpatient department and resumes his self-administered IV drip. He receives another phone call from the woman. Her voice is despairing yet calm. 'My father died. What now?'

That was at Wuhan's darkest moment. Even months later Lin is reluctant to recall that scene. 'Watching patients die without being able to help them, we doctors ...' He chokes up. 'We really were completely useless.'

*

During that endless spring, Lin Qingchuan signs many death certificates. Some stipulate 'cremate immediately'. In most cases, he fills the section for cause of death with 'respiratory failure', 'myocardial infarction' or similar. Very few cases mention 'pneumonia' or 'pulmonary infection'.

In January, Lin had received an instruction from 'higher up': no mention of pneumonia can be made on death certificates. This instruction is relayed by telephone, probably to prevent any document from being leaked. The government has set up an epidemic information network connected to each hospital for the primary purpose of collecting statistics on infections and deaths. On 11 February, Lin sees an order on his hospital's WeChat group instructing doctors who issue death certificates to 'verify the situation'; according to the order, if the name of the deceased is not included on the government's epidemic information network, the cause of death must not be recorded as pneumonia. Part of the instruction comes with exclamation marks: 'In the extraordinary period, great care must be taken when attributing death to pneumonia or pulmonary infection on death certificates!! If there is a history of other diseases, then record the other diseases as cause of death!'

During sleepless nights, Lin Qingchuan sees corpses growing cold and hears heart-wrenching wails.

With the explosive increase of infections, the already-small supplies of goods and medicines dry up. One morning, Lin sends his social media group a photo of a misshapen face mask. 'This is the face mask that has been with me for a week. Today it will be honourably discharged. Don't worry, our supplies are adequate, and our pharmacy still has zero-zero-zero-zero boxes of anti-inflammatory drugs.'

People cannot be treated due to the serious shortage of medical supplies, and some become hysterical. They are coughing phlegm all over the hospital lobby, perhaps deliberately coughing on others or smearing their saliva and sputum all over the place. A few even announce they will go to crowded areas to spread the virus. 'They were either despairing or crazy, and many were on the brink of complete breakdown,' says Lin.

After infusing the five packs of levofloxacin, Lin's symptoms improve but he still coughs often and his chest hurts. Moreover, the point of pain keeps moving about. 'Sometimes it was in the hilum, sometimes it was in the upper left lung.' On 30 January, he rushes over to the Wuhan Pu'ai Hospital hoping to get a CT scan, but there are too many people in front of him and he gives up.

Many doctors and nurses are 'battling the virus while sick', and without support. 'They treat patients during the day and treat themselves after hours ... The government said it would provide transportation for doctors and nurses, but in fact it was impossible to find a vehicle. They also said hotels would be provided,' he says contemptuously, 'but it was all empty talk.'

Two young nurses make a deep impression on Lin. Their home is over six kilometres from the hospital. To get to work on time they set off on foot before dawn, and at the end of the day they plod home. 'Those nurses were pitiful,' says Lin. 'Their monthly salary was only 601 RMB [renminbi or yuan, equivalent to A$123] but their return journey was a dozen kilometres, and that's as the crow flies.'

In Lin Qingchuan's hospital, and in all Chinese hospitals, such low salaries for nurses are common. Their plight is just part of life. They are usually contract workers or temporary hires. They do the most dangerous and arduous work for meagre salaries. In a difficult situation, they frequently substitute shifts, working twenty-four hours straight or even longer, and then have a few days off. Their exhausting work schedules make them more susceptible to infection. On WeChat, Lin often writes things like: 'Today another young nurse got infected. So sad.'

On 7 February, the night of wailing, there is an outpouring of deep sympathy among the citizens of Wuhan for the young whistleblower Dr Li Wenliang, for what he had to endure and his tragic death from the novel coronavirus. Lin's dry cough returns and there is a dull ache in his chest. He thinks of Li Wenliang and emotions well up. He writes on social media:

In this city under siege
Hero is a tragic word
...
My colleagues die
I see no light
And hear no sound
Everyone silently awaits their fate
...

The saviour of the people
Is not a doctor
Nor is it medicine

*

Lin Qingchuan was born in the 1970s and is unmarried. In his small hospital, with three Communist Party secretaries and two directors, he is a key member of the medical team. His friends see him as optimistic, strong and with a sense of humour. But now he frequently sheds tears for the desperate people with nowhere to go. He cries for the sobbing and pleading he hears on the phone and for heartfelt donations from the public.

As he leaves the outpatient department on the cold night of 27 January, Lin sees a tramp in distress. He is bundled in tattered cotton wadding, huddled in the middle of the road. Lin takes his temperature and gives him a physical check. He is motionless, weakly moaning, 'Cold, cold, cold ...'

No one knows the man's name or where he comes from. He wears glasses and perhaps has read many books. On that cold night, he is an insoluble problem. Lin makes several phone calls, but no hospital is willing to treat the man and no aid station is willing to take him in. In the end, all Lin can do is hand him over to the neighbourhood security guard. 'I never saw him again and I don't know whether he lived.'

Three days later, Lin Qingchuan encounters a lost cat named Three Flowers. Probably less than a year old with a little bell around her neck, she looks with pleading eyes at passers-by, miaowing as if asking for help. Lin makes a home for Three Flowers out of a cardboard box and every day brings something for her to eat. He often talks about her with his friends, telling them that she is pregnant and how adorable she is, like a father speaking about his little girl.

On 9 February, Lin is transferred from the community hospital to a very busy isolation station, where sick patients are separated from the public. He has no time to look after Three Flowers and doesn't know where the poor little creature ended up. She has probably died. In that miserable spring, many pets die in Wuhan, at home or on the streets. No one cares.

Lin has to work twenty-four-hour shifts at the isolation station every three days. He likens the station to a funnel: 'When hospitals couldn't accommodate the large number of fever patients, they were sent here. As soon as a bed became available at the hospital, we sent the most critically ill patients back to the hospital.' Owing to the lack of medicine and the ban on treatment at the isolation station, Lin is limited to giving check-ups, taking temperatures and doing his best to offer comfort. The station leader instructs Lin Qingchuan as such: 'You have to comfort the patients to ensure their emotional stability.'

On 13 February a patient returns to the isolation station. She has begun to feel itchy all over and her throat is swelling. Lin Qingchuan does a preliminary examination and realises she is having an acute allergic reaction to the medicine she's been given. He rushes downstairs to tell the station's leadership and requests a vehicle to take her to a hospital emergency department. The leader of the isolation station is a Communist Party propaganda officer. He asks Lin, 'Can she go there by herself?'

Lin replies that she can't and the situation is so critical, she might die at any moment. The leader looks at him sternly: 'Give me something in writing.'

Lin finds a pen and paper and furiously scrawls an explanation. The leader glances at it, frowns and says, 'I can't read this. Use a computer.'

Lin runs over to a desk, types his explanation into the computer, prints it out and hands the printout to the leader. The leader reads it, unhurriedly picks up his telephone and proceeds to ask his own leader for instructions. 'Hello, I've, er, got a situation here ...' Lin overhears the reply: 'Matters like this are not my responsibility, right?'

Lin is burning with anxiety. He says to his leader and to his leader's leader, 'It's a simple matter. Just send a vehicle. The hospital is close, at most it'll take five minutes to send her there.'

But it isn't really a simple matter. Late that evening, Lin fretfully checks the patient's situation – 'Doctor, I can't breathe.' He's dumbstruck as the leaders shirk their responsibilities, from one phone call to another and then yet more phone calls: section chief to director; director to department secretary; layer upon layer of leaders like nested matryoshka dolls. They have enormous authority but are unable to solve simple problems. Finally the leader in front of him hands over a few sheets of paper and says, 'We have discussed the matter. Follow the instructions in this document.'

Lin Qingchuan examines the document, about to burst into tears. 'They kicked the ball back and forth for an hour and it all came back to the starting point: the doctors shall be responsible for on-the-spot issues and the leadership will handle arrangement of a vehicle.'

This patient is lucky. During that hour of countless phone calls, her body overcomes the allergy; the swelling in her throat retreats and her breathing returns to normal. Shaken, Lin returns the document to the leader, saying, 'Forget it, not needed.'

'No one dared take responsibility,' says Lin, shaking his head. 'They'd rather let a patient die than put their signature on a document because as soon as they sign off they are responsible. In the end it means no one dares make a decision.'

Lin takes to his social media page to express his indignation: 'In our eyes, people's lives come first; in their eyes, people are just balls to be kicked about.' While this Kafkaesque story reveals how the Chinese government works, Communist Party propaganda will boast about 'the superiority of our system' and how this superior system helps China to defeat the virus. But that patient almost died from their superior system. This superior system allowed a controllable epidemic to become a calamitous once-in-one-hundred-years global pandemic.

Lin's isolation station is a dull grey building – a hastily repurposed hotel. All the windows are sealed and several security officers guard the tightly locked main entrance. In a car outside the station, a senior leader sits nonchalantly, and in the command centre further on, the big boss looks like he's on holiday. In the two months he works there, Lin Qingchuan enters the command centre only on that one occasion. Officials there sit, legs crossed, sipping tea. 'That's what they called the front line,' says Lin sarcastically.

These leaders know nothing about medicine and have almost no contact with patients, yet they decide if people can come or go, live or die. Later, many of them are promoted and receive awards, but Lin Qingchuan, who works twenty-four-hour shifts while sick, receives nothing.

The isolation station has over one hundred beds and is often full. Most admissions are later diagnosed with the novel coronavirus, but some are isolated for different causes. Lin sees a young woman with a high fever who has been in isolation for about a week. She is later diagnosed with chickenpox. It takes the leaders two full days to agree to discharge her. 'You locked me up here,' says the young woman, 'but what if I had become infected with coronavirus?' She is furious. 'If I'd died, would you take responsibility?'

The station has no sterilisation equipment and no partitioning between dirty zones and isolation zones. Doctors, nurses, orderlies and patients are crowded together, breathing the stale and contaminated air. Lin is issued with one set of PPE for each shift, so he wears his protective equipment while eating, washing and going to the toilet. He wears it walking up five floors and back down again because the lifts are reserved for patients. When he goes on his rounds to each room, he has to lift up his mask to check the patients' conditions and talk to them face to face. In Lin's mind he is like a chipped jar – being a bit more chipped won't make much difference. 'There was no other way, as I was already infected. If I really got …' He shakes his head. 'Then I would have deserved it.'

At the end of each day's work, Lin Qingchuan is completely exhausted, so tired that he doesn't feel like talking. The exhaustion also means he can't get better. On 17 February, he has another X-ray. The infection has moved from the lower part of his right lung to the middle of his right lung. He prescribes himself another three packs of levofloxacin. Later he sounds guilty when he talks about it, as if being able to survive is shameful: 'My hospital only had a tiny amount of medicine, just enough to save ourselves.'

On 7 March, as the Wuhan government tries to implement 'gratitude education' to encourage people to express thanks to the Communist Party for its leadership in fighting the virus outbreak, Lin Qingchuan meets an ambulance driver. Mr Zhang is in his fifties. After Wuhan was locked down, he drove there from another province without telling his family and became a volunteer in Lin's hospital. In the next month, he busily drove several thousand kilometres around the streets of Wuhan, ferrying hundreds of patients, including critically ill ones. To avoid cross infection, he usually slept in his car. On 6 March, a tumour had been found on Mr Zhang's lung.

Lin and his colleagues arrange for treatment and start a collection which quickly exceeds 30,000 RMB (A$6100). They take the donations to Mr Zhang but he firmly refuses to accept because he 'didn't want to bring any trouble to Wuhan'. Lin is deeply moved. 'Facing Zhang, I felt so ashamed. Ashamed and humbled.'

Eight months later, Mr Zhang will die at home. 'I thought his condition was not too bad. Never would have thought ...' Lin writes on WeChat. 'I cried.'

In those seventy-six days of torment, many people like Mr Zhang quietly left home and did their best to help the people of Wuhan despite the risks. Then, without clamouring for fame or recognition, they quietly went home to live their lives, disappearing into obscurity. They have no seats of honour at the grand award ceremonies; in China, honours belong only to the leaders.

*

Lin Qingchuan has been a doctor for twenty years but still cannot understand the absurd protocols implemented during the disaster. In the isolation station, results of the nucleic acid tests are classified as secret documents. They are available to the security guards at the main entrance but not to the doctors. Lin occasionally asks the security guards about a particular patient's test results. The security guards act like the leaders: 'That's secret. Can't tell you.'

'It was chaos,' says Lin Qingchuan. 'Many patients did not have medical files with them. We had to search all over the place to find the information.' The doctors organised an 'internal nucleic acid sharing WeChat group'. Someone would search the internal hospital network then quietly share the findings with others, like a secret agent in a spy movie, furtively prying into state secrets that contain information on their patients' conditions.

What's more, Lin says, 'Nucleic acid tests are extremely inaccurate, while antibody tests are more reliable. They knew it, so why did we only do the nucleic acid tests and not test for antibodies?' Lin Qingchuan answers his own question: 'It was to make the numbers look better.'

In March, the government dispatches a new doctor to the isolation station. He occasionally looks in on patients but mostly communicates with Lin Qingchuan online. At this time the number of patients staying at the isolation station hovers around seventy. Lin sends medical files of recovered patients to the doctor, and with his agreement and the further approval of the leadership, the patients are released from isolation.

Lin has a good impression of the doctor because he is cautious and responsible. They work together to ensure some of the patients are able to return to their families. But with many patients still in isolation, the government is dissatisfied. The newspapers are energetically praising China's victory in the antivirus battle. According to the official narrative, from 18 March there are zero new cases (except for three days, each with one confirmed case), and people are eagerly waiting for the lockdown to be lifted. The government wants to fulfil people's expectations and make the numbers look good.

'They wanted us to kick patients out of the isolation station as soon as possible, the more the better,' says Lin Qingchuan. But he is clearheaded about the consequences of this approach and refuses to sign off, as does the new doctor. So the doctor is transferred away and replaced by two new people, one a radiologist and the other from some other department. This two-man squad is a so-called 'expert team'.

'I really have to admire them,' says Lin. 'They arrived at four in the afternoon, sat down and began to review X-rays of patients with lung infections. They said, "This one's shrunk," then picked up another X-ray, said, "This one's shrunk too," and so in a few short hours they kicked out over forty patients.' Lin watches the cavalier medical diagnoses. 'They still had lesions, their inflammation was not completely cured, and they were still infectious. That's scary.'

However, for the government the numbers still don't look good enough. Soon another expert team arrives, and a further twenty patients are sent home. Only the critically ill remain, the ones Lin Qingchuan calls the 'old catastrophe' cases. 'Their symptoms were obvious. Surely, you'd feel embarrassed to discharge them too, right?'

But the government is unconcerned about embarrassment, so they send another three-person team. Lin never sees them because he is off duty for two days, but when he returns to work on the third day he finds that all the old catastrophes have been sent home. The isolation station has not a single patient. He sighs helplessly. On social media he reminds his friends: 'Some horror patients, highly contagious patients, have been set free. You'd best patiently stay at home.'

Lin calls these dangerous practices a 'political cure'. He writes on social media, 'When medical issues are politicised, we'll never be free from fear and a normal society will be far away.'

The isolation station closes. Lin Qingchuan returns to work at the small hospital, but he is panicky. He knows that this kind of 'political cure' will bring disastrous results. And sure enough, four days later, the isolation station reopens, and the patients who have been discharged are hauled back in again.

That's just a few days before the scheduled lifting of Wuhan's lockdown. The city's cherry blossoms have long withered. The newspapers claim there have been no new cases for many days. The high praise becomes ever more resounding. Every leader is quivering with excitement in preparation to welcome the great victory.

Lin Qingchuan knows the good news is not true. 'The isolation station reopened, which goes to show that the virus had bounced back. In fact, after those patients returned home, they would have infected many others, infecting their whole family.' He repeatedly says, 'Infecting their whole family.'

Lin believes people who died at home or didn't present to hospitals 'were most likely excluded from government statistics. Take my own case. I was definitely infected but did not have an official diagnosis, so I was not included ... Among us doctors, I reckon not a single one believes the government numbers, they're just false.'

After the lockdown ends on 8 April, the streets of Wuhan gradually return to life. The citizens begin to go out and shop as before. Sometimes even laughter can be heard. But the wounds deep in the hearts of many people remain raw and difficult to heal. 'I often cry at the drop of a hat,' a woman writes on a WeChat post. Many can empathise.

Even on the streets, few believe government case statistics. 'At least twice as many,' says a young person disparagingly. 'Since when was this government ever honest?' People who wholeheartedly support the government are still guardedly sceptical about the fatality statistics. 'It should be more than two thousand,' says a shopkeeper. 'It was a chaotic situation so we should expect there to be a bit of discrepancy, right?'

Based on the number of community hospitals and death certificates that he signed, Lin estimates the real number of deaths at around sixteen times the official figure.

*

In May, Lin Qingchuan posts on WeChat several photographs of himself posing as a beggar. He's covering his face with both hands as he squats at the roadside. In front of him, he's placed a cardboard box in which there are a couple of coins. He writes: 'Today I'm not only begging for food for myself, but also for colleagues who are encountering difficulties.'

Lin Qingchuan's monthly salary is less than 3000 RMB (A$624). In a city like Wuhan, that's barely enough for the basics of life. But he hasn't been paid for several months. It's even worse for the nurses. While the virus is raging, doctors and nurses are called 'white-robed angels' in state media, but as soon as it is over no one asks the angels if they have eaten.

The community hospital is classified as a 'public welfare service provider'; the government pays for part of the salaries while the hospital raises the rest by charging patients. Over that endless spring, the doctors and nurses throw themselves into antivirus work, for which the hospitals do not charge, so Lin's hospital has almost no income at all and the government appropriations are persistently late. By May the hospital is in debt 3.6 million RMB (A$740,000) and on the brink of bankruptcy.

The Chinese healthcare system is of a complex and sinister design. Patients cannot afford to be sick, while doctors and nurses can barely eke out a dignified standard of living. Every hospital is a commercial enterprise in which a doctor's income is often based on how much medicine they sell and how many operations they perform. They are salespeople as well as doctors. Sometimes they are con artisits too. Many take bribes from patients – 'butchering the patients', as it's known, as if they are slaughtering livestock.

On 24 December 2019, as the virus silently spread among the populace of Wuhan, a relative of a patient in Beijing stabbed a doctor to death. Incidents like this occur across China because people are incensed by high fees and ineffective treatments. Many doctors die in knife attacks. Chinese newspapers and TV news programs denounce 'violent attackers' but rarely delve into how hopeless and angry these people feel, let alone mention the healthcare system that 'kills doctors'.

Lin's begging act is a kind of performance art. He is protesting at the government's incompetence and extravagance. Shortly before the epidemic exploded, Wuhan hosted the grand Military World Games. Many stadiums had been built, requiring an enormous workforce and 140 billion RMB (A$29 billion). Xi Jinping personally attended the opening ceremony and gave 'important instructions', saying that the 'military games are a display of China's image'. Several months later, Mr Xi's words sound like biting sarcasm.

That flashy sporting event generated almost no benefit, just adding to Wuhan's debts. For that reason, the shortages that follow are even more severe.

When the isolation station reopens, Lin Qingchuan is again caring for patients. By now, to celebrate the victory over the virus, the government has held many award ceremonies and presented innumerable trophies and merit certificates. Lin is constantly anxious, never shaking hands and always wearing a mask as soon as he leaves home. 'The more the government says nice-sounding things, the more nervous I become,' he says.

Lin is also unsettled by anti-scientific propaganda and agitation. There is a medical theory in China called 'traditional Chinese medicine'. TCM believes that the universe and the human body have identical structures, with both built from five mutually constraining and engendering elements – metal, wood, water, fire and earth. The heart is of the fire element, the kidneys the water element. The lungs of millions of people infected with coronavirus are metal.

Over a period of two thousand years, this medical tradition has turned into a complex and intricate form of mysticism. In recent times, many knowledgeable people have criticised TCM for being unscientific. But in China countless people, including Xi Jinping, believe in this 'wisdom of our ancestors'. Mr Xi frequently praises TCM, at home and abroad. In the eight years of his reign, this medical mysticism has been promoted as never before. In May 2020, Beijing publishes a draft law for public comment that virtually criminalises 'vilification or slandering TCM'.

During the global pandemic, the Chinese government continues to promote TCM. According to its White Paper published on 7 June, 'In Hubei province, more than 90 per cent of confirmed cases received TCM treatment that proved effective.'

Such statistics put Lin Qingchuan in a quandary. 'You can't say these numbers are incorrect. Every day many Chinese medicines were delivered to the isolation station. They wouldn't kill you and patients were permitted to take as much as they liked, so that statistic is correct because 90 per cent of the patients really did try Chinese medicine. But as to the therapeutic efficacy, only heaven knows the answer.'

He sees three kinds of traditional medicines at the isolation station, one of which has six ingredients, including orange peel, mulberry leaf and red root. Lin snorts disdainfully: 'Even the worst medical student would not use that stuff to prevent and combat a virus. It would be just as effective to burn some paper, mix the ash with water and drink it.' He writes some doggerel satirising these medicines.

Children's urine and black dog's blood
Drink it down and have no fear
Of pissing on your shoes, you hear.
You have science
I have magic
Bullshit all the way to Mars.

'The disaster is far from over,' Lin says. He's worried the virus will explode again. He's also concerned about a future economic depression. But what he fears most is China's political environment and the imminent threat to freedom. 'The Communist Party doesn't know how to tackle the virus, but it knows how to control people.'

In Wuhan's seventy-six-day lockdown, he personally experiences the power of the Party and the state. 'In the past we'd heard about urban grid management administrators, but we never saw them. During this pandemic, urban grid administrators overtly made their presence felt and I fear that in future it will be difficult to be free of them.'

The urban grid management administrators that Lin speaks of are an important component of the Chinese government's measures to control the masses. Neighbourhoods are divided into grids, each overseen by grid attendants wearing red armbands. Like tigers who never sleep, they constantly monitor the residents. During the pandemic their powers grow, and they become increasingly arrogant and unreasonable. On 16 April, two men wearing red armbands arrive at Lin Qingchuan's hospital claiming they have come to inspect 'the return to work and resumption of production'. A nurse tells them, 'We never stopped working.' It's a neutral answer, but it infuriates the two men, who swear rudely at the nurse and threaten to drag her off to the police station. Lin

Qingchuan intervenes. He feels indignant. 'How dare a "Red Armband" set the police on a nurse. Who does he think he is?'

Lin works at the isolation station until June. He is not sure if he is cured, but he stops coughing and he moves normally although when he is tired his chest hurts. He is a strong and humorous person, often laughing at work. But when he stops laughing, he can't help thinking of the tragic spring and the helpless patients who died.

The images often trigger tears to stream down his cheeks. For him, the experience of the spring of 2020 is a wound that will never heal. It will haunt him for the rest of his life.

In June, Lin Qingchuan writes on his social media page, 'Excuse me, leaders, would one of you please settle our outstanding salaries. We medical workers are waiting for our rice. Even slaves have to eat.'

2.

You want me to live, and I want you to live, too

Jin Feng trudges home, brooding on how to die.

Xia Bangxi is preparing to head off to his night shift, but as he is about to leave, his wife arrives. He senses something is wrong. After persistent questioning, Jin Feng finally reveals the truth: she is infected with the novel coronavirus. Jin Feng shoves her husband and their son Xia Lei out of the room, closes the door and silently sobs. She is still weighing up the best way to kill herself.

Xia Bangxi opens the door. 'The TV says this disease can be treated. Why not get it treated?'

'Just leave me alone,' snaps Jin Feng.

In that moment, Xia Bangxi reads her mind. 'Well, in that case,' he says, 'I'm not going to work.'

It is late on the evening of 29 January, the seventh day of Wuhan's lockdown. Jin Feng does not get a moment's sleep, and neither does Xia Bangxi, who paces back and forth at the doorway, keeping his eyes on his wife. Just before first light, he says to Jin Feng, 'Don't worry, I'll take care of everything.'

Sixty-four-year-old Jin Feng is a cleaner at the Wuhan Central Hospital. She heard of the virus early on, in the hospital elevators and the doctors' changing room – an infectious disease in Wuhan that is much more severe than SARS. 'That scared me,' says Jin Feng, 'so I always wore a mask at work.'

At the time, the Chinese government wasn't worried about the disease – it was more concerned about preventing panic – so doctors were forbidden to wear protective equipment. A cleaner like Jin Feng is even less eligible for protective equipment.

Although she has worked at the hospital for over two years, she is not officially a member of staff. She is employed by a property management company called Pearl River Management. A typical 'indispensable redundant person', she mops floors, disposes of rubbish, and even cleans the doctors' surgical clothes and shoes, which are often bloodstained and soiled. In two years, she has encountered many doctors and nurses, though few of them know her name.

On 29 January, Jin Feng had worked from early in the morning until the evening, cleaning many rooms on many floors, sprinkling disinfectant in every corner. Close to the end of her shift she began to feel uncomfortable: 'Feverish and weak all over.' She went downstairs to register at the outpatient department, had blood drawn for a test, and was given a CT scan, which she handed over to a nurse.

The nurse examined the scan and confidently told her: 'It's very likely you're infected. You should see a doctor straightaway.' Jin Feng works at the Nanjing Road unit of the Wuhan Central Hospital. During the pandemic it's responsible for diagnosis only, so for treatment she would have to go almost seven kilometres to the Houhu branch.

By this time, it is after 10 pm and the lobby of the hospital is overflowing with fever patients. Jin Feng slowly walks outside into empty streets. The whole city is deserted, like a village submerged by a flood. 'Forget it,' she thinks. 'I won't go for treatment.'

Suicide is not an easy choice, but on that evening of 29 January, Jin Feng is unable to come up with a better way out. 'This disease is so infectious,' Jin Feng says to herself. 'I'm over sixty. Many people have not been cured, so why would I want treatment?' She cannot afford the cost of treatment anyway, and she can't possibly isolate in her own home. 'I didn't want to hurt my family,' she says. 'I did not want to infect them.'

No. 22 Poyang Street is in the centre of Wuhan, just metres from the banks of the Yangtze River. It is the dormitory compound of the Wuhan Central Hospital, with scores of old, dilapidated, dusty apartments. The peeling walls are mottled with small advertisements for fake IDs and toilet-unblocking services. The air reeks of sewage, stews and rotting food. Piles of hexagonal briquettes sit like clusters of poisonous mushrooms.

This is where Jin Feng and her family live. They share the apartment with another family – a shared kitchen, a shared toilet, and jet-black concrete floor. 'How could I possibly isolate in a place like this? That's why I thought it would be better to die. If I were dead, they would be safe.'

Only when Xia Bangxi deploys all his persuasive powers does his wife relinquish thoughts of suicide.

When dawn breaks on 30 January, Jin Feng telephones her superior – a woman surnamed Yuan – to ask for help. 'I work in the hospital too,' says Jin Feng. 'I just hope the hospital could help me.' Ms Yuan tells her, 'Just go. When you get there, someone will treat you.'

Xia Lei remembers none of this and has no ability to help his parents. A 2007 car accident left him with a severe head injury. Now forty, his intellect is more or less that of a primary school student. His memory is worse. He can barely remember anything, and he has great difficulty clearly uttering a complete sentence. When Jin Feng is interviewed, Xia Lei quietly sits to one side, listening to his mother recount past miseries, occasional contributing by muttering, 'This fucking disease, so ferocious.'

At 10 am, the neighbourhood committee dispatches a vehicle to take Jin Feng, Xia Bangxi and two other infected people to the branch hospital in the Houhu district. They are greeted by the huge 'infected persons marketplace' – a long line of infectious people queuing up for treatment, some seated, more just lying on the ground. The lobby is cacophonous with people running around, shouting. A constant stream of vehicles for transporting corpses is coming and going, and family members are wailing piteously. Not far from Jin Feng, a tall, strong young man is on his knees begging a doctor to treat a relative. 'So many people were dying,' says Jin Feng. 'Even the doctors were helpless.'

The two people who arrive with Jin Feng have 'good connections' at the hospital, so they are promptly allocated beds. But Jin Feng is just a lowly cleaner unworthy of such privileged treatment. 'No doctor called us,' says a person in charge, 'so how can you prove you work at the hospital?' When Xia Bangxi begs for his wife, the response is cold: 'You say you're with the hospital, he also says he's with the hospital. How do I know if you really are with the hospital?'

Jin Feng has a high fever and can barely sit upright. Xia Bangxi holds her in an embrace, while Jin Feng telephones Ms Yuan again. She responds, 'I've already called the leadership of the hospital. If they don't make arrangements, what else can I do?' Jin Feng asks, 'What should I do now?' Ms Yuan replies, 'Nothing, just wait for notification.'

Notification never comes. Jin Feng has no alternative other than to huddle into her husband and follow the flow of people inching forward. They eventually register, have all sorts of check-ups, then sit in the corridor and wait for an IV infusion. They are famished but cannot leave the hospital until 2 am.

It's a freezing winter's night. There are no taxis, and neither the police nor the hospital can possibly arrange for a car to shuttle them home. Jin Feng and Xia Bangxi instead have to share a rented bicycle. Every ten minutes or so, a frail Jin Feng has to stop and rest for a while. Then Xia Bangxi lifts her back onto the bike and the two of them, clinging together and faint from lack of food, pedal through the bitter wind, slowly making their way home.

That is the first day. Then follows the second day and the third day ... Each morning, to arrive at the hospital as early as possible, Xia Bangxi rises at 4 am, cooks rice porridge for Jin Feng and attends to her until she finishes it. They pack a simple lunch for two, a bottle of milk and a piece of fruit. Then they ride the bike, stopping and starting, gasping for breath all the way to the hospital. It is less than seven kilometres, but it often takes them more than three hours to get there. After arriving at the hospital, they join the queue, shuffling forward for five or six hours just for the chance of an IV infusion. For Xia Bangxi this is a perilous routine, but he doesn't mind because he has vowed to get his wife cured. 'Don't worry,' he says to Jin Feng. 'Even if I get infected, I will use my life to save yours.'

While they edge forward in the treatment queue, Dr Li Wenliang dies in the very same hospital. Jin Feng and Xia Bangxi see the flood of journalists arriving and the floral wreaths piling up at the main entrance, but they don't pay much attention and have no idea about the repercussions of Li Wenliang's death for China and the world. They are preoccupied with their own survival.

On that evening of 7 February, many people die silently. Nameless and only numbered, they are covered in white cloth and reduced to piles of grey powder.

As Jin Feng waits for treatment again in the sprawling 'infected persons marketplace', Xia Bangxi is by her side, ready to lend an arm to support her. With bloodshot eyes, he occasionally coughs behind his face masks. 'I don't know how he became infected with this disease,' says Jin Feng. 'He had been very careful. He wore a plastic raincoat and three masks. How could he get infected?'

Xia Bangxi's sickness comes on fast and feverishly. By 9 February he is vomiting blood, yet he still forces himself to rise at 4 am and cook rice porridge for Jin Feng, before together they head off to the hospital.

They are given nucleic acid tests. Jin Feng is negative. Xia Bangxi tests positive, but there are still no beds available at the hospital. After IV infusions, they struggle to get back home. 'At that time, I really couldn't walk, and neither could he,' says Jin Feng. 'I had no other options, I had to go to the neighbourhood committee.'

No. 22 Poyang Street is an area particularly hard-hit by the epidemic. Red stickers declaring 'fever household' are everywhere; every building has at least one infected person inside. Jin Feng hears there are 226 doctors and nurses infected at the Nanjing Road unit of her workplace. The number of deaths is unknown but at least five people of professorial rank are among them.

After the epidemic explodes, the Chinese government seizes the opportunity to strengthen its rule. No sick person is permitted to obtain treatment on their own; treatment decisions are to be made by a grassroots level of the government, that is, the neighbourhood committee. The committees are now responsible for collating infection statistics, distributing food, arranging transportation – everything. On the evening of 9 February, when Jin Feng carries Xia Bangxi, vomiting blood, into the neighbourhood committee office, no one takes any interest. A leader tells them: 'It's too late to do anything today. Come back tomorrow.'

The next day is cold, overcast and raining. Xia Lei lugs his father down the staircase, then Jin Feng supports him back to the neighbourhood committee. What she sees pushes her into despair. 'As soon as they saw us, they ran away,' says Jin Feng. 'They all went into hiding … Only one person remained.'

There is a yellow demarcation line outside the neighbourhood committee office which Jin Feng and Xia Bangxi have no right to cross. As they stand shivering in the rain, Xia Bangxi coughs violently, occasionally spraying blood. Jin Feng moves a chair and helps him sit under the eaves, but he doesn't have the strength to sit. 'I set him down, but he just slid off the chair.'

Jin Feng begs the remaining neighbourhood committee member: 'Just look at my old man,' she says. 'He's vomiting blood. I beg you. Please save him.'

Like other Communist Party organisations, the neighbourhood committee excels at avoiding responsibility during the pandemic. 'Doesn't matter what you say,' says Jin Feng, 'they have all sorts of excuses. They just didn't want to take us to hospital.' The neighbourhood committee will not report Xia Bangxi's name to the higher authority as he cannot produce a nucleic acid test report. He cannot produce the report because the hospital had notified him by telephone. There is no report.

The back and forth of begging and refusing continues unabated for hours. At noon the committee finally agrees to arrange a car to take Jin Feng to a hotel and Xia Bangxi to an isolation station. 'That was not a place for treating the disease,' says Jin Feng. 'They sent us into isolation. He was so sick, but they didn't arrange for treatment. They just sent him into isolation.'

Xia Bangxi's condition worsens at the isolation station. Jin Feng telephones many times from the hotel. She hears his weak voice say there is no one looking after people, let alone treating them. There is no water and no food. 'They keep us here,' he gasps, 'just to let us die.'

Jin Feng is frantic. She calls the neighbourhood committee again. They tell her: 'It's none of our business. Your husband is at the isolation station, so talk to the doctor there.' It takes several hours to get through to the doctor. He responds: 'We don't have any medicine here and we're forbidden to treat patients, so you'd best speak to the neighbourhood committee.'

The desperate and the helpless are trapped in a system from which there is no escape. Jin Feng begins to contact every relative, every friend, begging them to phone the mayor, the neighbourhood committee, the media, every organisation with any power. She feels the weight of these calls like a mountain, yet they are not enough to have her husband admitted to hospital.

At the time, the government had vowed to treat every single novel coronavirus patient, but due to inadequate medical resources, many people like Xia Bangxi are abandoned to await death. They die at home or in the corridors of hospitals or simply on the streets of the city of despair.

Jin Feng thinks of her husband's vow to care for her and the unforgettable words he uttered: 'I will use my life to save yours.' She can't hold her tears back. Throughout that wintery night, with the desolate sound of rain falling, Jin Feng weeps as she desperately makes telephone calls. In the isolation station on the other side of the city, her husband is dying.

At noon the next day, Jin Feng leaves her isolation hotel, gasping for breath as she rushes to the neighbourhood committee office. She sinks to her knees and howls at the officers: 'Why didn't you report our names to the higher authority? It wouldn't have cost you a penny. You just had to say the word. Why couldn't you do that?' She then asks, 'Do you have parents? Do you have children? Did you not report our names because we are peasants?'

Someone responds: 'Didn't you say you want to sue? Well go ahead.'

Several months later, when Jin Feng recalls that scene, her fury is unabated. 'I was still sick then, kneeling down, short of breath. I couldn't stop the tears. I just wanted to die.'

Xia Lei has also not completely forgotten the scene. 'Those fuckers just watched Mum kneeling there.'

Scenes like this never appear on Chinese TV. In that bitter spring, apart from Jin Feng and Xia Lei, no one remembers a sixty-four-year-old woman kneeling on the muddy ground, crying and begging for this world to save her husband. She really did think about dying. 'If you don't send my husband to hospital,' she wails, 'I will die here, I'll die here in front of your eyes.'

At 4 pm on 11 February, the neighbourhood committee finally reports their names to the higher authority and dispatches a van to take Jin Feng to the isolation station so she can take her husband to hospital.

By then, Xia Bangxi's strength is almost completely depleted. He strains to get to the van's door; he flops over the seat but doesn't have the energy to pull himself into it. Jin Feng crouches behind him, holds his legs in her arms and uses her shoulder to push from behind. Slowly, she heaves him into his seat, then goes to the other side of the van to get in herself. Hugging her husband tightly, she uses all her strength to hold him upright.

'You want me to live,' she speaks close to her husband's ear. 'I want you to live, too.'

*

Xia Bangxi was born in 1953; he is the same age as Xi Jinping. When Xia Bangxi was twenty-six, a matchmaker introduced him to Jin Feng. Soon the couple married. Like many marriages of the time, love blossomed little by little under the arduous circumstances of life. Together they planted rice, cotton and sweet potatoes, and raised chickens, ducks and pigs. Jin Feng still remembers them transplanting seedlings and threshing grain. ‘Our crops were pretty good,’ she recalls. ‘Sometimes we’d work through the night to be sure the daytime work was not delayed.’ It was an era of extreme poverty. They rented a leaky hovel, where the landlord’s coffin was stored in the doorway to be sure of a dignified burial. After Xia Lei was born, they built their own home, brick by brick.

While always poor, the family was warm and harmonious. Xia Lei never saw his parents fight or get angry. ‘The old man and the old lady were pretty good tempered,’ he says. Jin Feng never mentions the word ‘love’ as she explains, slightly embarrassed, ‘We were husband and wife for forty-one years and he always looked after me well.’

Their hometown was about sixty kilometres from Wuhan in a small village called Dragon King’s Watchtower. The village consists of a few dozen old houses, some unoccupied, battered by the elements and slowly falling apart. Xia Bangxi spent most of his life in this village. For over twenty years he was the village Party branch secretary. He always smiled warmly, doing his best to help everyone.

Jin Feng is a high school graduate, which in the era of Mao Zedong was an extraordinary achievement. Naturally, she became a schoolteacher, in a shabby village school where she taught for more than twenty years. Some of her students made it to university and one even went to America, something that makes her very proud. She breaks into a radiant smile. 'Those kids were really smart.'

In official documents, Jin Feng is merely a locally funded non-government schoolteacher. The term 'non-government-employed teacher' is one of those abstruse terms that means Jin Feng is 'not a teacher' or is a 'temporary teacher', so she has no possibility of promotion and cannot enjoy the benefits a teacher in the city enjoys, like a retirement pension and medical insurance. Around 2002, this 'temporary teacher' of twenty-two years was dismissed. The compensation was paltry but Jin Feng doesn't complain; she even feels it's what she deserved: 'The new teachers are young and educated, so I'm not really qualified.'

After she was fired, Jin Feng worked in the fields for about a year. The exhaustion was unbearable. 'I'm short. The rice stalks I carried were as tall as me.'

That was when Xia Lei was in the serious car crash. The medical fees left this already humble family completely broke.

Jin Feng had to give up farming and head to the city to get menial work – dishwashing, cleaning – because the pay was slightly better than farm work. As she aged, her income declined. In 2014 her salary was 3100 RMB (A$670); in 2017, 2600 RMB; and in 2018 when, at the age of sixty-two, she was hired as a sanitation worker responsible for cleaning the contaminated operating theatre, her monthly salary was 2250 RMB.

When he reached fifty, Xia Bangxi had been dismissed from his position as Party secretary. He received an allowance but it was small, almost nothing, so to make ends meet he had to follow his wife to the city. His diabetes meant he could not do any heavy work, so right up until Jin Feng was infected he worked as a night guard, making 2600 RMB (A$530) a month.

Like most Chinese people, Jin Feng and her family bear the injustice of their lives with equanimity. They don't complain and are rarely angry. They simply work diligently and draw strength from every small kindness that comes their way. In 2016, Jin Feng was a dishwasher at a Sichuan restaurant. When her mother died she asked the boss for two weeks off. He didn't dock her pay when she returned. She was deeply moved. 'That boss was such a good person,' she says. 'I'm truly grateful to him.'

While the family resides in Wuhan, their household registry records them as peasants. They are in the city as 'migrant workers', which in the language of communist China means they are second-class citizens. Yet they accept the situation. They still worship the Party and believe in the Chinese government, using the honorifics

Chairman Mao and Chairman Xi when referring to Mao Zedong and Xi Jinping. They are full of praise for the government's handling of the pandemic. 'The government's policy to my mother is alright,' says Xia Lei. 'But for my father ...' The dissatisfaction is directed at the neighbourhood committee because they 'did not properly implement the Party's policies'.

*

Xia Lei doesn't get to see his father as death closes in. At dusk on 11 February, the van takes Xia Bangxi to the Hankou Hospital. Several doctors and nurses push him in a wheelchair into an operating theatre. Jin Feng watches, brimming with hope and with thanks. 'I was so grateful to those doctors. In such a dangerous situation, they worked at saving my old man,' she says softly. 'I wholeheartedly hope they can live to one hundred.'

The next morning, Jin Feng sneaks into the operating theatre. She sees her husband, eyes shut, lying motionless on a hospital bed. She walks over to the bed and touches his forehead, then gently grasps his hand. Xia Bangxi can barely open his eyes. Jin Feng tells him, 'Don't lose heart, in the hospital there's a chance to be saved.'

Xia Bangxi's lips tremble as he speaks, almost inaudibly. 'You must take care of yourself. You are sick too. You have to eat properly.'

Her tears stream but Jin Feng dares not cry out loud. Choking with emotion, she tries to encourage her husband, just like she had encouraged her students in the classroom years ago. 'Have confidence, the doctors will surely cure you.'

Xia Bangxi takes his wife's hand, speaking a last sentence with difficulty. 'Go and get a nutritional injection ...'

Jin Feng barely sleeps the following night. In another part of the hospital, she ruminates on the forty-one years of joys and hardships that she and Xia Bangxi have been through together. Soon after 5 am on 13 February, before it is light, a doctor hands her a 'critically ill notification'. Her spirits sink. After two more hours, several doctors and nurses come out of the operating theatre. One doctor tells her: 'Xia Bangxi couldn't be saved. He has died.'

Jin Feng does not know how to describe her feelings at that time. 'It was like the city walls collapsed,' she sobs, anguish in her eyes.

Over the next three days, all Jin Feng can do is cry. She does not eat a grain of rice. She herself is deemed no longer critically ill and is finally allocated a two-person room in the Hankou Hospital. To avoid disturbing her roommate, she weeps silently on her bed. 'I had only one thought – to go with my old man. I didn't want to live.'

The hospital sends people to console her, and even allocates two psychologists. They sit by Jin Feng's bed saying, 'The disaster is nationwide. Many people have been infected and many have died, not just your husband.' And of course, they mention the Party. 'The Party and government are very concerned and take the matter seriously ...'

As Jin Feng is sinking to the depths of grief, Wuhan's cherry blossoms bloom and then wilt. It's the most beautiful season, so perhaps Xia Lei, again at home alone, watches petals floating about, though he won't remember them to tell his mother.

'It's so very difficult, not just a little bit difficult,' says Jin Feng later, as she looks at Xia Lei by the window. It's hard for Xia Lei to go shopping because making transactions with his mobile phone confuses him. Once, as he tried to buy a bottle of alcohol, the shopkeeper stared at the cash in his hand with horror and threw him out of the shop. 'The son of a bitch wouldn't take my money!'

Jin Feng sighs and says in a soft voice, 'If it weren't for the neighbours' help, he would never have survived.'

On 5 March, Jin Feng is declared cured and is moved to one of the temporary hospitals known as 'mobile cabin hospitals' for fourteen days of quarantine. This kind of hospital is an 'important invention' of the Chinese government during the pandemic. It's not really a hospital but more like a huge warehouse, with men on one side and women on the other, a total of two hundred beds. Jin Feng thinks it is fine – the other inmates are very nice, and the food is good. 'Three meals a day, including fish and meat.' Sometimes songs break out, like 'Without the Communist Party, There Would Be No New China' and 'Socialism Is Great', and happy patients begin to dance gracefully. Jin Feng joins in a few times, but on each occasion she soon retires. 'There were lots of families, husbands and wives, brothers and sisters,' she says. 'When I looked at them, I would always think of my old man.'

Jin Feng often dreams of Xia Bangxi. In her dreams the world is always beautiful, and there is no coronavirus. One day she and Xia Bangxi are walking along a street holding hands. It seems like they are out shopping. Xia Bangxi asks her, 'Did you bring enough money?' Jin Feng says she did; her pockets are stuffed full of money. Then they come to a street stall and Jin Feng puts her hand in her pocket to get the money but pulls out a blank piece of paper. She tries again and another blank piece of paper comes out.

She wakes up crying. In those days she spends almost every night crying in her dreams. The other patients, woken by her sobbing, gather around to comfort her. 'My old man wants to speak to me,' she tells fellow inmates. 'I never burnt ghost money for him, so he wants me to give him money.'

'I feel he hasn't left me,' says Jin Feng later. 'Sometimes when I'm doing something, I suddenly turn my head to see if he's by my side.'

Jin Feng completes her fourteen days of isolation on 19 March and is shuttled home in a vehicle dispatched by her neighbourhood committee. She puffs as she climbs the stairs and opens the door. Xia Lei is standing inside the doorway.

'You're back at last,' he says, then bursts into tears.

Jin Feng is in a daze as she looks at her son. Emotions well up and she doesn't know what to say. Leaning against a wall for support, she begins to cry with him.

*

After she leaves the temporary hospital, Jin Feng must home-isolate for fourteen days more. The illness leaves her with severe long-term effects. Her whole body frequently aches, she has ringing in her ears, and she has difficulty raising her hands over her head. The doctor says her organs are damaged.

The neighbourhood lockdowns remain in force, so she has to rely on Xia Lei to go out for groceries. This child with the face of an adult often gets lost and buys the wrong things – fatty meat instead of lean meat, potatoes instead of cucumbers. But Jin Feng is consoled because he seems free of worries. He's always happy.

The neighbourhood committee begins to bombard Jin Feng with phone calls urging her to collect Xia Bangxi's ashes from the funeral parlour. She is disgusted. 'What did you do when he was alive? When he needed treatment, you ran as far away as you could go. Now he's dead, why have you become so concerned for him?'

'My old man's death was so unjust,' says Jin Feng. 'If they had not sent him into isolation and instead sent him to hospital earlier, he may not have died.' She pauses for a moment, then adds, 'What they're worried about is that I'll start wrangling.'

In China, after each disaster the state media asserts in a nonchalant tone, 'The family members of the deceased are emotionally stable,' as if death is a trifle and the family members are without feelings. In truth, a tumult of blood and tears bubbles like molten rock beneath a mountain. In the aftermath of the Wuhan disaster, the government uses bribery, threats, surveillance and arrests to ensure the grieving and angry do not protest. The neighbourhood committee delivers food and gently beseeches Jin Feng to collect her husband's ashes and bury them. The government provides 3000 RMB (A$630) consolation money for every coronavirus victim, but when Jin Feng demands the money, every day for a week the committee responds: 'You have to bury the ashes first, then you can get the money.' By taking the consolation money she would be acknowledging Xia Bangxi's death, indemnifying the government and relinquishing her right to seek redress. 'The family members of the deceased are emotionally stable.'

By 3 April she can no longer resist the entreaties and threats of the neighbourhood committee and goes to collect Xia Bangxi's ashes. 'I didn't want to wrangle with them, I just didn't have the energy,' says Jin Feng. 'Besides, being lenient to others is actually being lenient to yourself, so I let it go.'

The Hankou funeral parlour has many different kinds of cremation boxes. Jin Feng chooses a white one because she thinks white is pretty. There is no photo on the box, just Xia Bangxi's date of birth and date of death. Red fabric is wrapped around the box and yellow tassels are sewn onto four sides. Jin Feng likes the red fabric. She embraces the box as she slowly walks out of the funeral parlour. 'In all those years together, that was the first time I could hold him up,' she later says.

Jin Feng can't afford a grave plot in the city. She instead takes her husband back to their home village to bury him in the fields they had tilled together. In any case, she knows the city is not their real home and she will eventually return to the village so that Xia Bangxi can see her at any time.

Xia Bangxi's mother still lives in the village. She's over ninety and Jin Feng is afraid to tell her of her son's death, out of concern her aged body would not withstand the sorrow.

The fields they tilled have been left fallow for years and are covered with waist-high weeds. Jin Feng selects a hillock for the burial. During the pandemic, funerals are simple affairs – no burning of ghost money and no religious ceremonies. The villagers are fearful that Jin Feng could be carrying the virus and deny her entry to the village itself, and will not even allow her to participate in the funeral. So while Jin Feng sits in a car nearby, Xia Lei places the cremation box in the grave and the villagers help him fill the grave with dirt. Village leaders speak a few words to memorialise Xia Bangxi's impoverished but hardworking life as their Party secretary. Xia Lei mutely observes, not really understanding the proceedings.

Xia Bangxi's grave does not have a tombstone. In accordance with local custom, tombstones for people who die an inauspicious death are erected only after three years. Jin Feng wonders whether she'll still be alive then.

A few days later, Jin Feng dreams of her husband again. In the dream, Xia Bangxi is healthy and handsome. He knows Jin Feng likes to play mahjongg and says to her, 'You can go and play.' But she doesn't want to go because she wants to be with her husband. Xia Bangxi smiles and gives her a little push. 'You must be exhausted. Go, go have some fun.'

Jin Feng wakes up. She sees the wall of their apartment, blackened with soot from the stove, and herself, tiny in the boundless night. She can't help sobbing silently. 'I know what he meant. He hoped I would live on happily,' she says to herself.

*

After Wuhan's lockdown is lifted, several journalists come to interview Jin Feng. On the way, they buy some food at a McDonald's. For the journalists it's nothing special, but Jin Feng's is such a frugal family, rarely eating out. Xia Lei is extremely excited. 'Today I'm enjoying an exotic delicacy,' says Xia Lei. 'In my forty years, this is my first time to eat McDonald's.'

The journalists have rented a car to take Jin Feng and Xia Lei to Xia Bangxi's grave. It is raining heavily, so they have to slog through muddy fields to light fireworks and burn ghost money in the rain. Jin Feng kneels in front of the small pile of earth howling hoarsely, 'My old man. You have abandoned me ... Old man, I want to go with you.'

The citizen journalist Zhang Zhan has also been told about Jin Feng. She visits her on 17 April. Touched by Jin Feng's story, Zhang telephones Pearl River Management, and in no time several leaders arrive to give Jin Feng 2000 RMB (A$420) in consolation money. They promise not to dock her wages and tell her she should go back to work as soon as possible. Jin Feng is hesitant. 'If I go back to work, they will have an excuse to fire me, right? I'm old and unwell. If a tiny mistake was made ...'

Jin Feng and Xia Lei live in Wuhan for four more months. By August, Jin Feng can no longer afford the rent and decides to move back to their hometown. Xia Lei helps his mother pack up their old quilts, their tattered clothing, a few pieces of well-used furniture and some cooking essentials. They rent a van to take their ragged possessions to their hometown, hoping to survive in the most frugal way. 'We have no choice. After my illness I can't work, and there's no way we can survive in Wuhan,' Jin Feng sighs. 'We have no choice. We have no choice.'

Over Jin Feng's life of toil, hardship has never been far away. As a girl sixty years ago, she experienced starvation during the tragedy of the Great Famine. As she grows older, she worries that a terrible famine might return. In that long Wuhan spring, she often wanted to die, but she struggled on. 'Future' is a beautiful word, but for Jin Feng, it's an extravagance for which she has no use. 'What future can someone like me have?' she asks. 'I no longer have the strength to live on.' Her hope is that the government will issue Xia Lei with a disability certificate. Her son would then be able to live on after she dies.

She pauses and sighs for a long time. 'I know it's not easy, I know.'

3.

I drive forwards, but the wind blows back

'Gotta survive,' says Li as he dismounts at an intersection. 'If it weren't for that, who'd want to take people on a motorcycle at a time like this.'

On the roads near the Hankou Railway Station, Li is unobtrusive. He's short and thin. He wears a hat to keep warm but also to hide his face. If you happen to walk close enough you'll see that, beneath the brim of his hat, the face is perpetually alert and vigilant.

Li is one of Wuhan's 'black' motorcycle operators who transport people illegally. During that unrelenting spring of 2020 he straddled his motorcycle to carry doctors, nurses and coronavirus patients along the highways and backstreets of Wuhan. 'From the start of the lockdown til the end,' Li says, evincing a certain degree of pride,

'I was out on my motorcycle every day. I didn't ever stop working.'

Li is now in his sixties. He was born in a small village outside Wuhan. After graduating from high school, he moved with his family to Wuhan city and they set up a wonton stall. At the time, the business was neither legal nor illegal. They had to continue paying the village a 'migrant work fee' of around 60 RMB (A$12) a month; this payment allowed them to leave the village legally but it didn't mean they could legally enter the city. They had to be wary of interactions with the city's authorities – the police and the chengguan (the local government by-law enforcement officers), as well as anyone connected with the government. They could suddenly appear in front of the stall. Sometimes they'd accept a little cash; that was the gentle treatment. The not-so-gentle treatment meant being cursed, beaten and chased away, or having the stall overturned and their woks, bowls and stove smashed.

Around 1980, Li abandoned the family's wonton business to be a trishaw driver in Hanzheng Street. In more recent years, Hanzheng Street has become famous for shopping malls selling commodities from clothes to electronic devices. In Li's day, it was a chaotic, raucous open-air market with narrow, muddy streets and dilapidated buildings. In the torrid heat of Wuhan summers, the shirtless young Li furiously pedalled his trishaw through this scene, revealing his less-than-impressive arms and chest, sweating profusely as he hauled merchandise for traders. 'In those days I had a licence,' says Li, 'a legal licence the government issued to me.'

In 1992, the Wuhan city government banned trishaws. Li received 6000 RMB (A$1200) compensation, ending his career as a trishaw driver – the only licensed business he has ever had. Wuhan was redeveloping and Li quickly found an opening as a demolition contractor. He enlisted workers from the countryside who wielded sledgehammers and crowbars to knock down buildings. He then sold whatever he could salvage from the rubble. The work was dangerous. Without any protective equipment to speak of, injuries and deaths were common. But the income was good, and Li became wealthy. He also became addicted to gambling. 'I didn't make friends with the right sort of people,' Li explains. 'Someone took me to a casino. At first, it was just small-scale and I thought it was fun. Later I lost control, betting more and more, and losing more and more.'

From 1992 to 2012, Li gambled heavily, even visiting Macau, where he boozed, gambled and did some things he'd prefer not to talk about. He blew several million RMB. This less-than-noble life changed everything. His demolition business went downhill so far he had to shut it down. His wife wanted a divorce, which he agreed to, though they didn't sever relations. They still live in the same neighbourhood and Li provides her with living expenses on a regular basis. Prior to the coronavirus catastrophe, Li proposed to his ex-wife. She didn't accept the proposal, but she didn't reject it either. She just said 'more observation needed', to be sure he had really given up the evil of gambling. And of his son, Li says, 'We used to be very close, but because of my gambling habit ...' He sighs. 'I can't blame him, I brought it all on myself.'

After the demolition business closed, Li worked for a while installing windows, doors and pipes in new apartments. He was over fifty, the work was hard and the pay was only just enough to cover living expenses. He applied for several credit cards, borrowed against each card in succession and repaid in succession, like a mini Ponzi scheme. He used the money to gamble, hoping to change his fortunes, but his debts just piled up. 'I was too clever for my own good,' he sighs ruefully. 'Credit cards are really bad.'

Around 2016, his boss, a former employee, fired him. Li didn't hesitate for long; his age and his savings balance didn't allow hesitation. 'I was old and no longer able to do hard manual labour. I could be a janitor, but the pay is too low.' He says it again: 'Gotta survive.' Instead Li bought a second-hand electric motorcycle for about 1000 RMB (A$200). Now he heads to the streets near the railway station and stays alert and hopeful as he sizes up every passer-by.

'I've seen big money and also the wider world,' says Li, exuding self-satisfaction, revelling in his glory days of debauchery. But in an instant, he sighs again, complaining he was possessed by the devil. 'The money was already in my hands and just like that I gave it all away. Now, at this age, I have to drive a motorcycle taxi. To tell the truth, I'm pretty miserable.'

Most of Li's passengers are peasants who work in the city. They do not want to take the exorbitantly priced taxis but, being unfamiliar with the streets, they are willing to risk hiring an illegal motorcycle taxi. Li's profession does not put much emphasis on honesty. Usually, he quotes a high price, say 20 RMB (A$4). People who know what the price should be will complain, 'How come these two wheels cost more than four wheels?' Then they lower the price to eight or ten yuan. If Li doesn't object, the passenger sits astride the back seat and, holding Li's shoulders, they bounce their way into the city. None of the passengers ask for a safety helmet, and anyway, Li himself doesn't wear one. As far as he's concerned, safety is not particularly important. 'Gotta survive.'

In China, every business must have a government-issued licence, including writers, artists and performers, with Li himself being an exception. He doesn't even have a driver's licence, which would be a big headache because the government does an annual assessment – and of course there's a fee. Li doesn't want to pay, and in any event, he'd never pass the test.

Although Li has lived in Wuhan for forty-three years, he is still not a legal Wuhan resident. His household registration is still in his old village, and his rural retirement pension has in recent years been about 300 RMB (A$61) a month. 'That small amount is not enough to do anything in Wuhan.' But he is grateful to the government. 'The policy is good because in the past there was nothing.'

Before the catastrophe in 2020, Li made over 100 RMB (A$21) a day, an income he relied on to buy the necessities of life, to provide financial assistance to his ex-wife, and to pay off his debts. The government does not approve of Li's business and has established a squad dedicated to confiscating motorcycle taxis. If nothing out of the ordinary happens, the squad nabs Li around once every three months. They seize his motorcycle and issue a penalty notice: 'Operating an illegal business, fine 3000 RMB' (A$610). Li just ignores the penalty. 'Three thousand RMB,' says Li, followed by a profanity, 'is enough to buy two motorcycles. Why should I pay the fine?'

When the squad doesn't receive the fine, they sell the seized motorcycle to a 'connected' company, which repaints the motorcycle, spruces it up and on-sells it back to Li and his fellow motorcycle taxi drivers. In four years,

Li has bought a dozen or so motorcycles, some of which may well have been his, though he can't be certain. 'One or two looked familiar, yet there was something different.'

When Li was young, he watched the movie *Railroad Guerrilla*. This film is the Communist Party bragging about itself, telling the story of a bunch of miners and drifters who, under the leadership of the Communist Party, roam the railway lines like Robin Hoods, mounting sneak attacks on the Japanese invaders and their supplies, achieving ever greater victories.

Decades later, Li views himself as a guerrilla. Though he never initiates conflicts, he conceals himself like a mouse stealing into a cat's lair, dodging the authorities while riding along Wuhan's avenues and alleys, always on the lookout for the fearsome police and shrewd motorcycle snatch squads. 'I'm illegal, my motorcycle's illegal,' he says with a hearty laugh. He falls silent for a moment, then says in a low voice, 'The law ... I just don't get it.'

Li hears about a novel coronavirus early on, at least he thinks he did. His residence is not far from the Huanan Seafood Market, which, according to the Chinese government's earliest explanations, is the source of the virus. Before November 2019, he and his fellow motorcycle taxi drivers frequently ferried merchants from the market, occasionally helping them transport goods like fish, shrimp and crabs as well as all sorts of wild animals. He doesn't recall ever transporting bats and he doubts anyone eats them. 'Bats are disgusting. Who'd eat 'em?' he says. 'Anyway, I've never seen that.'

Around the middle of November, one of Li's colleagues was 'taken away for treatment'. Li says Wang was quite old, about seventy-eight. 'He was once a soldier and had been running a motorcycle taxi for over thirty years near the Huanan Seafood Market. After he was taken to hospital, we assumed he had been infected with the virus,' says Li. 'Don't know what happened to him; maybe he was cured, but if he wasn't cured, he's most likely dead by now.'

There's a large blank space in Li's memory. He doesn't remember how the city descended step by step into panic. He doesn't remember what he did in the following months. 'Riding my motorcycle, eating, sleeping,' he recounts slowly. 'Nothing particularly exciting.'

At this time the novel coronavirus is stealthily spreading throughout China and then to the whole world. Li is oblivious to these developments, just riding his second-hand motorcycle taxi from home to the railway station and then all over the city. His passengers must have included infected people, but Li is not afraid and never wears a mask. 'The passengers sat behind me, so as I drove forwards, the wind blew back.' Li has a karmic view of life. 'If I was meant to get infected, there's no hiding from a virus, right?'

Just before the Spring Festival, or Lunar New Year, Li returns to his home village where his parents are buried. Chinese custom requires him to sweep their graves. He buys some ghost money which he burns in front of their graves and makes a wish that his parents protect him in the coming year.

That is 22 January, the day before the Wuhan lockdown. Li has not heard the news about the lockdown and has no idea how bad the situation is. Rather than spend the night in his hometown, he travels overnight back to the dangerous city. Unlike the millions of residents trapped in Wuhan, Li feels extremely fortunate. 'I was almost stuck in my hometown. There's nothing there. What would I eat? Or drink? Luckily, I came back,' he says. 'Coming back, I could survive.'

*

At 2 am on 23 January, Wuhan authorities promulgate the lockdown order, or as the media gently puts it, 'Wuhan is pressing the pause button.' Millions of people panic. Within twenty-four hours, five million leave the city, coinciding with the coldest weather on the central plains of China. To fight off the cold, Li covers the motorcycle seat with a thick brown woollen jacket and wears colourful padded cotton gloves. He also starts to wear a mask as he rides to the railway station. A cold misty rain drifts from the sky. People are shouting and running about like ants facing a flood.

At about ten in the morning, just when the lockdown order comes into force, Li sees a middle-aged woman in black. She stands in the station entrance, holding a wheelie suitcase in her right hand and a light-blue umbrella in her left. Her dishevelled hair and bewildered look are those of a little girl who can't find her way home.

Wuhan's lockdown, so significant for the whole world, for Li only means a woman in black in the midst of a vast sea of people with her wheelie suitcase and light-blue umbrella. 'She was working as a nanny in Wuhan and wanted to go home for the Spring Festival. By that time, it was impossible to leave the city, so she asked me to take her to a place to stay. I took her around for half an hour but couldn't find an open hotel. She asked if she could stay at my place, but I said no. Later she asked me to buy her a blanket so she could sleep in an underpass.'

Li doesn't know how that woman survived the lockdown. 'There were a lot of people like that who couldn't return home, or got off a train at the wrong station; so many, uncountable.'

On the next day, Lunar New Year's Eve, Li sets out as usual. Another driver tells him there are no customers at the train station – it is all happening at the hospitals. Li rides his old motorcycle to Houhu Hospital, where he sees the raucous 'infected person's market' and the long line of people at the hospital entrance. He makes dozens of return trips, transporting some patients home and more to the hospital. He could hear them sitting behind him wheezing, coughing and groaning, but he maintains he wasn't afraid because there's no use being afraid.

Li spends that night at his son's house with his ex-wife and their one-and-a-half-year-old grandson. The fractured family is finally reunited. They cook dumplings, fry up several dishes, and even watch the New Year's Gala on CCTV. Li has not forgotten what he witnessed at the hospital entrance – the pain and hopelessness, the wailing, coughing and moaning – but he can't help being enchanted by the dazzling song and dance performances. At about 8.40 pm, six immaculately dressed presenters appear on stage. Using their skills at rousing emotion, they recite in unison a poem titled 'Love Is a Bridge'. The poem praises 'Secretary General Xi Jinping's series of instructions', mentions 'the Party Central Committee' twice, and invokes 'love' innumerable times. 'Please believe in China, everything will be better!' And then they declaim with great passion, 'Love is the best bridge. Step on it, Wuhan!'

Li is deeply moved by this not-so-poetic poem. 'Well written, well delivered. I felt the whole country's concern for Wuhan. Really moving.'

But the slogans of the presenters are of no help to Li. Nor are Xi Jinping and the Party Central Committee.

Every day, Li continues to ride his old motorcycle to hospitals looking for passengers.

He is jealous of two colleagues. One has connections in the Hubei Cancer Hospital and is hired as a temporary worker. He wears PPE while spraying disinfectant all over the hospital. The work only lasts about two weeks but the daily pay is 600 RMB (A$120). Li is astonished. 'Six hundred! But without connections you can never get that.'

The other colleague picks up an old infected patient at a hospital entrance for a trip of less than one kilometre. The old man pays 100 RMB (A$21). Li knows a job like that is not as straightforward as it appears. 'The old man could not walk on his own, so my colleague had to get him home and carry him upstairs, which was not easy.' And yet Li envies him. 'It was a little risky, but the money was easy.'

When the lockdown begins, the motorcycle taxi business takes a big hit. Around the Hankou station, only five drivers stay on the job. Li knows every one of them. It's hard for them all but Li feels his own circumstances are the most miserable. 'They all had savings, so it was no problem for them to stop working. Just not me.' He shakes his head, perhaps recalling his dissolute days. 'Can't blame others, it's all my own doing.'

At least for Li, business is healthy. 'There were hardly any vehicles on the road, no buses, no taxis, but there was a demand, right? People needed to visit their parents, visit the doctor, buy medicine, and there were infected people too weak to walk. None of them tried to bargain. Whatever price I quoted, that was the price. They even said to me, you're risking your life to do motorcycle taxi business.'

Perhaps because he feels guilty, Li is unwilling to say how much he earned during that time. He knows he is engaged in an illegal business. He stammers his defence. 'This work I do is for the greater good, right? ... Yes, I did receive money, but I helped them, right? ... Speaking from the heart, if it weren't for me, what would have become of them?'

Working from 9 am to 7 pm, Li carries twenty to thirty rides a day. The majority are infected with the coronavirus, though he does transport the occasional volunteer, nurse or doctor. On 30 January, he meets a couple in their sixties. Li takes them from Wuhan Central Hospital to Jiangwan Road. The husband holds on to Li's shoulders while the wife squeezes behind her husband and holds on to his waist. They discuss the coronavirus catastrophe and life under lockdown. About two days later Li receives a phone call. It is the husband. 'We both tested positive,' he says. 'Terribly sorry, driver, you'll need to get tested.'

Li doesn't follow the advice. From the beginning to the end Li never gets tested. He repeatedly claims he is 'not scared' because 'that is a feeling he never gets'. But sometimes he reveals the real reason: 'The virus is frightening, but no food to eat is even more frightening.

'My family is very scared. My wife, my son, they don't want me riding the motorcycle. They say, life is important. What happens if you get infected? My son lost his temper at me. I know they want what's good for me, to be honest,' confides Li. 'The pressure was huge. If I had money, what would it matter if I didn't go out for a few days?'

He does try to protect himself. 'I wore a mask, I wore gloves, I did my best to avoid taking cash; as soon as the passengers left, I disinfected. Gotta survive,' he sighs.

On those dangerous rides, Li sees all sorts of people, but he is only willing to talk about the ones he charged a standard fare or from whom he took no money at all, like one woman from Jiangsu province. 'Young, less than twenty. Told me she wanted to go to Taibei Road to be a volunteer. I ask her, "Aren't you frightened?" She replies, "There are times when people are needed." I really admired her, so I didn't charge her much.'

One experience is bizarre. Around 16 February, Li delivers a patient home. On the way back to Wuhan Central Hospital, he hears someone call out from the window of a building overlooking the road. 'It was a man about thirty, really thin, with an ashen face. He asked me: "Will the police arrest me for being out during the lockdown, will I go to jail?" I told him he wouldn't be jailed but might be dragged off to quarantine isolation.'

The ashen-faced man ignores Li's warning and executes a hair-raising leap from the second floor to the road, then sits on the back of Li's motorcycle. Li drives to an apartment block on Sanyang Road. The man sends a WeChat message, then a package is dropped out of a window. The man picks it up and gets back on Li's motorcycle. 'He didn't pay anything,' says Li. 'He said he'd pay me via WeChat but after I delivered him back home, he didn't come out again. What could I do? I couldn't start a fight with him.'

Li thinks the man was a drug addict. He doesn't like him but is sympathetic. 'Addiction to drugs and addiction to gambling are almost the same. Once you're hooked, you can't stop. In those days, they were having a hard time too.'

On 5 February, Li bumps into a regular customer. He is sixty-three with severe coronavirus symptoms. He is only two years older than Li, but Li usually calls him 'old man'. The old man does not live far from Li's place, in the Hongguang neighbourhood. Li picks him up each morning to take him to Houhu Hospital and watches him join the long queue. His customer doesn't exit the hospital until eight or nine at night. 'I took the old man to get an injection every day at over 2000 RMB [A$400] a shot, but it didn't help him. I took him there daily for three days, but I could see him get sicker by the day.' Li points to his throat. 'In the end this collapsed, and he couldn't talk or walk.'

On 7 February, Li delivers the old man home for what will be the last time. He pays double, then reminds Li in a weak voice, 'You must come again tomorrow morning.'

That night is Wuhan's night of wailing. As Li gets home, some citizens are blowing whistles, others are shouting from their windows. Li hears the whistling and shouting and sees the beams of light from mobile phones but is not particularly moved. 'So many people locked up at home are certain to feel depressed. They let off steam by shouting a bit. As for me, I don't think about it much. I eat when I need to eat and sleep when I need to sleep. Normal life,' he says. 'My mental state is pretty good.'

The next morning, Li rides to the Hongguang neighbourhood but there is no sign of the old man. He waits a while, but he does not see him or get a phone call. Li doesn't think much of it at the time. In that spring, missed appointments are not a big deal. Most bookings fall through.

A few days later, when he hears that someone has died in the Hongguang neighbourhood, Li immediately thinks of the old man. 'I think it was him,' Li says slowly, with a trace of sadness on his face. 'The old man paid for two trips.'

*

As far as Li is concerned, Wuhan under lockdown is a better world. No traffic cops, no 'squads', and everyone is generous. He rides down main roads, running red lights at will, the whole city his oyster.

On 11 February, while riding near Moon Lake Bridge, he encounters a police officer on duty. Li suddenly has the urge to play a prank on her. He rides up to her and strikes up a conversation with a hint of being provocative. 'Comrade officer, may I ask ...' The policewoman steps back, her eyes glaring wide, then shouts at him, 'I don't know, I don't know.'

Li laughs his heart out. 'I just wanted to give it a try, but I gave her such a fright,' he says, gesticulating wildly. 'Usually when we see a policeman we try to hide. I never thought I'd live to see the day when we could scare *them*.'

On 15 February, Li's golden days come to an end. Wuhan begins to lock down neighbourhoods strictly. Millions of people are trapped in their own homes. Every daily activity – grocery shopping, visiting a doctor, even birth and death – is handled by the local authorities. This kind of totalitarian epidemic prevention might protect some people, but it does not solve Li's food problem. 'What happens when you have no money?'

He finds chinks to exploit, like jumping over walls or sneaking out under the eyes of the guards. 'I'm a wily old fox who will always find a way out,' says Li. On the streets, he hardly ever sees anyone, but he always finds customers; that is to say, customers can always find him.

Around this time, a woman gets on his motorcycle. 'She was in her forties. Her mother was over eighty and very ill. It was impossible then to go to a hospital, there was no way to buy medicines and there was no one looking after her mother. She says, "Driver, I beg you, please take me to her."'

Li takes her from Xinhe village to Xiangheli. She is extremely grateful. She holds on to his shoulder as she tells him how difficult life is in isolation. 'If I don't go, what would become of my mother,' she says. 'She's over eighty, how many years does she still have?'

'It really was difficult for her,' Li sighs sorrowfully. 'She has a child here and a sick mother over there but can only handle one place at a time. If she hadn't found me, she would never have been able to go. It was a real long way. Walking would have taken her forever.'

A few days later, Li finds a 'legal' way to get out of the neighbourhood. He gets his ex-wife to go to a meal delivery platform – You Hungry? – and fill in some forms to register as a deliverer. 'I was too old for anyone to want me, but she's young enough to deliver food.'

Every morning, Li gets his ex-wife to scan her face for facial recognition confirmation to log on to the platform, then she accepts a delivery order. She gives it to

Li, who puts on the blue jacket issued to food deliverers and brazenly walks out of the neighbourhood. He then drives to the restaurant to pick up the meal and make the delivery. Some of the orders are quite easy but some require him to travel six or seven kilometres or even further. Li can't complain. 'Ten RMB an order, so five or six orders was fifty or sixty RMB. The customers were accommodating and didn't complain if the delivery was a little late. Quite nice, really.'

Li is vexed by the procedure for checking and verifying identity. After a few orders, the platform checks their information on delivery personnel, such as confirming they are wearing a mask. 'And the face scan was required to confirm the right person was working.' Li's counter strategy is to 'shoot through after making three deliveries'.

'That way they'd never catch me,' he says, sounding immensely proud of himself. 'I did that for several months without getting caught.'

Li still goes to Houhu Hospital often, mostly to pick up and drop off patients. On 7 March, Wuhan's Party Secretary Wang Zhonglin delivers the 'gratitude' speech, insisting citizens should 'express gratitude to the Secretary General, to the Communist Party' for their response to the crisis. About two days later, Li receives an order to deliver flowers to the hospital, a bunch of fresh flowers costing about 200 RMB (A$42). The attached message reads: 'Please make a deep bow to Dr Li Wenliang on my behalf.' Li arrives at the hospital entrance and respectfully lays the flowers on the stone steps. He hesitates a moment. He does not bow but has a heavy heart. 'Just pitiful,' he laments.

When Wuhan's weather turns warmer after March, with cherry blossoms piling up like snow on the branches, Li continues to ride his old motorcycle, shuttling back and forth through a city long gone to seed. He transports patients and delivers food but never once pays attention to the scenery by the roadside. 'Cherry blossoms? Why would I look at them? Can't survive on cherry blossoms.'

One day in the middle of March, Li is in Tangjiadun to pick up a 'girl who operated an internet shop'. She makes a deep impression on Li. 'Her home is in Yichang and she ran a small business in Wuhan. I could tell at once she's a hard-working girl. She dressed simply and worked late every night.'

Li is not skilled at describing people's appearances; he only remembers that the girl's Chinese zodiac sign is the rabbit – so she's either thirty-three or twenty-one years old. She sells items in hot demand from her internet shop: masks, gloves, disinfectant.

The first time Li sees her, she's preparing a consignment for the Hanyang Sports Centre. It's the longest trip Li makes during the lockdown, twenty kilometres. 'I delivered her there and she wanted me to collect her, but I didn't have enough charge left so I had to go home to change motorcycles. On the way back, the police at Moon Lake Bridge wouldn't let me pass. I called her and she began to walk back as we spoke. She walked about ten kilometres before we met up again. By then she could barely walk.'

Not long after that, the girl runs into even bigger trouble. The son of an official in the Health Commission tells her he has connections and can get his hands on some government-issue masks. She pays 40,000 RMB (A$8200) in advance. In the end she only receives 20,000 RMB worth of merchandise. Despite her repeated demands, he just won't deliver any more goods. He taunts her: 'Sue me.'

'She called me again to take her to the Health Commission. Officials there said it had nothing to do with them. She then wanted to go to the police, so I took her to the local police station, but they said it was not within their jurisdiction and suggested she go to the sub-bureau. The sub-bureau said, "Do you know what's going on now? You think we have time for such things? Go to a local police station."

'So I take her around for a few days but there are no results. She then said she wants to stage a protest outside the Health Commission. Guess what the police said? "This is a civil dispute. You can go to court, but don't cause a public disturbance because that constitutes obstruction of government administration, and that's illegal, you understand?"'

Li is indignant. 'That's unfair. How could she go to court and sue? The courts were not even operating then.' He shakes his head. 'Poor girl. She just wanted to make a bit of money and was cheated out of twenty thousand. And there was nowhere she could complain.'

Li often takes pity on others, and sometimes takes pity on himself. If you talk to him about that painful spring, of the tragic people and events, he frankly admits the girl's losses are not really worth mentioning. 'Yep, her case was not the most tragic,' he says. 'She's still alive.'

On the last day of March, Li encounters a person who is deaf and mute. His home village is about 100 kilometres from Wuhan. His mother has died there, and he is heading back for the funeral. He arrives at Wuhan station in a mad rush. Li remembers his anxious state. 'His hair was a mess, his face was unwashed, and he only had 220 RMB on him.' But he didn't have the correct certificate to enter the station. 'He's unable to speak so he was just pacing back and forth.'

Li walks up and asks if he wants to take his motorcycle taxi. The man takes out his mobile phone and types. He wants to know if Li can take him to find a hotel. By then the lockdown is easing and some small hotels are furtively reopening. Li finds one that charges 70 RMB a day. The next day Li meets up with him again. 'He wanted to go to the train station, but he couldn't get in without a certificate from the Civil Affairs Bureau. The

Civil Affairs Bureau told him to go to the Labour Bureau. I telephoned the Labour Bureau, which said they could issue a certificate, but he'd need documentation from his work unit.

'He didn't work in Wuhan so how can he get a certificate from his work unit?' Li recalls angrily.

Li looks on the man and takes pity, while the latter regards Li pleadingly, hovering around like the surveyor outside the castle in Kafka's novel *The Castle*. Unlike the novel's protagonist, K, this Chinese K is stuck inside the castle; no matter how many certificates he acquires, certification of certificates is still required, and he can never leave the castle.

Li writes a few words on the man's mobile phone: 'Do you trust me?' Mr K answers, 'Yes.' Li writes, 'Don't bother with BS certificates. Get on my motorcycle and I'll find a way to get you out of Wuhan.'

Mr K holds on to Li's shoulders as Li takes him to find a 'black' taxi driver called Qin Qin. Like Li, Qin is also engaged in illegal business, but at a higher level – he has a car. During the lockdown he is like a cunning smuggler, spiriting many people out of Wuhan. Li has no idea which road he uses, or perhaps he just doesn't want to say. 'You can still take back roads,' says Li, 'otherwise just shove some money in the officer's hands. After March, the controls were not so strict. If you really wanted to get out, there was always a way.'

By this time Mr K has only 150 RMB (A$30) left, but Qin Qin wants 600–1000 RMB. Li explains Mr K's situation. Qin hesitates for a while, then says, 'Forget about payment. He's disabled, his mother has died; I won't charge him.'

'I didn't take a penny and Qin Qin didn't either,' says Li. 'We are illegal operators, but we helped him big time.'

Li has never read Kafka, but he likes the story about the castle. He understands the travails of the surveyor, up against opaque bureaucrats, and also understands the obstacles on the road to the castle because it is just like China. He does not think the surveyor's difficulties insoluble. 'If there had been a black motorcycle taxi in the story,' he says gesticulating, 'every problem would have been solved.'

After the lockdown is lifted on 8 April, many residents ecstatically venture outdoors, like prisoners released after a long confinement. Li, however, once again falls into despair. His food delivery career is over because more and more people are entering the ranks. 'There's no way I can compete with them,' says Li.

As before, he leaves home at 9 am and hangs out around the Hankou Railway Station all day. But it's hard to find customers. 'Business is worse than before the outbreak. I'm lucky to make a few dozen yuan a day,' says Li. 'Even taxis have no business, let alone people like me.'

Li's WeChat account is called 'Only You'. The sentiment is probably directed at his ex-wife. He only sends one message to his circle of friends; it includes three photographs. One is a picture of a tree growing on an overhanging cliff with a caption reading, 'If you choose to plummet to the depths, no god can save you. If you are determined to live, you will survive even in the most desperate circumstances.' This is intended to show his ex-wife that he will never gamble again. She doesn't entirely believe him, and neither does he. When there are no customers, he reminisces – half in regret, half fondly – of the days long ago, when he was young and lived a life of debauchery. They were the best of times and the worst times.

Another photograph shows him at the Hankou Railway Station in 2018. Li no longer recalls who took the shot. He looks younger, while riding a different old motorcycle. The third photo shows a group of ants pushing a rock. The caption reads: 'When you march towards your goal, the entire world will make way for you.'

Li cherishes the memory of the days of the lockdown, the time when the pandemic was causing devastation, with millions of people suffering and angry. It was actually his happiest time. 'Illegal, risky, but quite happy.' After a long moment of silence, he finally admits he was also scared – scared of the virus. He feared getting ill and dying but he had no choice. 'What else could I do?'

he asks rhetorically, answering, 'Work a day, live a day. When you die, then you're dead.'

As for the future, Li has no plans. 'At my age, I won't be able to find other work. I'll just keep on riding a motorcycle taxi until I can't. Then I'll do whatever I can.'

'And then?'

He suddenly begins to laugh. 'There is no then.' He laughs again and tugs on the brim of his hat, covering half of his face. 'There is no then.'

4.

A man who wants to pursue the light

It's the day before the Lunar New Year, 24 January, and Liu Xiaoxiao spends the night alone. He eats dumplings and watches the New Year's Gala on CCTV. He particularly likes a song called 'New Year's Disco' in which the Hong Kong singer William Chan, in a red costume, sings and dances with his two partners on a glittering gold stage. They sing, 'These are the best of times, these are beloved times,' followed by, 'You must never forget, you are Chinese forever, no matter where you are.'

'New Year's Disco' is a happy song celebrating high-speed trains, 5G and the internet economy, tacitly praising the Communist Party's rule. But Liu Xiaoxiao is unable to be cheery. He is worried about the epidemic in Wuhan.

Several months later he still recalls the day when more than eight hundred people became infected with the novel coronavirus and twenty-six died. 'The numbers are doubling every day. What the hell will happen next?'

Liu Xiaoxiao is thirty-four years old and works as a substitute teacher at the No. 4 Middle School in Wujiashan, a Wuhan subdistrict. In the month before the Spring Festival, he was still teaching. Despite a large number of Wuhan residents becoming infected, he was completely unaware of the virus. He vaguely recalls that one day in December 2019 a kindergarten closed 'due to influenza' but classes quickly resumed. The government never provided an explanation, and simply instructed the school management to ensure ventilation. On the last day of 2019, Liu Xiaoxiao saw a news item on his phone announcing that twenty-seven cases of 'pneumonia of unknown cause' had been diagnosed in Wuhan but that the 'illness is preventable and controllable' so there was no need for the public to panic. On 19 January 2020, a government official still insists at a press conference that the novel coronavirus is 'not highly infectious' and the 'risk is low', so of course it is 'preventable and controllable'.

Like most Chinese people, Liu Xiaoxiao believes the news, despite it emanating from the state media. He reads about the Wuhan police 'dealing with' eight 'rumour mongers' 'according to the law', but quickly forgets about it. In the eight years since Xi Jinping's rise to power there have been so many news items like that. Every police station in the country is busy cracking down on 'rumours' – some are fake news, most are just criticism of the government. Practically no one pays attention to what rumour mongers actually say, and Liu Xiaoxiao doesn't either. The government tells him not to panic so he doesn't panic. He maintains his daily routine of teaching, tutoring and occasionally driving his car for an online ride-booking platform. Right up to 23 January, he is tutoring in a student's home without taking any precautions, and the student doesn't either.

That day, 23 January, is a day that shocks the world. At about 10 am, on the orders of Beijing, Wuhan's airport and train station are shut and all transportation in the city is halted. No one is permitted to enter or leave the city. Eleven million people are now confined to a huge jail.

While Wuhan residents sink into dread and grief, on television people in Beijing are cheering and singing for the CCTV New Year's Gala. A Wuhan shopkeeper says, 'When I saw Jackie Chan sing, "Does my country look sick?" you know what I thought? I felt' – he then curses profanely – 'I felt I had been abandoned, abandoned by this country. I felt we had all been abandoned.'

On the day of Wuhan's lockdown, Liu Xiaoxiao leaves the city and returns to the place of his birth. Anlu is a small town, 110 kilometres from Wuhan, where his father Liu Shiyu is living in a nursing home. Traditionally, the Spring Festival is a time for family gatherings, so he must visit his father.

Liu Xiaoxiao describes his journey home as a 'thriller'. He sets off at dusk. It's bitterly cold and almost no one is outdoors in Wuhan; his headlights peer through the curtain of rain onto the empty streets. The city appears to have been dead for a long time. The freeways are closed, but smart people are always able to find a 'back door' around China's laws and regulations. Under the cover of darkness, he drives frantically down a small secondary road that the police have not yet sealed off. Eventually, he finds a way to Anlu.

There's never been a shortage of sick people in Liu Xiaoxiao's life. When he was eighteen, his mother was diagnosed with leukaemia. After a few days in hospital, she decided to cease treatment; she wanted to save the money for her son's university education. Forty days later, she died.

A year later, his father had a stroke and lost consciousness. Liu Shiyu's treatment cost over 50,000 RMB (A$10,200), bankrupting the family. Liu Xiaoxiao relied on assistance from his relatives and his school to scrape enough money together to pay off the cost of the operation. At that most difficult time, he had thoughts of jumping off a building.

After the operation, Liu Shiyu was left disabled. He had no feeling in the left side of his body and needed a wheelchair or a cane to get around slowly. Liu Xiaoxiao was then still at university. Unable to look after his father, he took him to a nursing home. Ten years later, Liu Shiyu looks like a skeleton.

Next was Lu Xue, Liu Xiaoxiao's lover. The story has a beautiful beginning. Girl falls in love with boy and, ignoring her family's opposition, elopes 500 kilometres to be with him in a place far from home. They live together happily for seven years, until 2013, when Lu Xue is diagnosed with colon cancer. Her family is penniless. She can only rely on Liu Xiaoxiao.

He takes her to hospital, where she undergoes chemotherapy and has much of her colon removed. He spends all his savings but it isn't enough. He pleads for help from friends and relatives and asks the media for assistance. A few newspapers and magazines publicise their story. There is a heartwarming photo of Xiaoxiao washing Lu Xue's feet. An episode of a melodramatic TV program even helps 'stage' their betrothal. All these efforts bring in some support, but it is like splashing a cup of water on the firestorm of Lu Xue's medical expenses.

Eventually, having exhausted every avenue, the destitute Liu Xiaoxiao leaves the hospital in despair. Lu Xue is even more despairing as she lies in a hospital bed awaiting death.

In China, few people can afford a serious illness. 'Diseases of the rich' like leukaemia and cancer might bankrupt a middle-class family, but for the poor they mean certain death.

Like most Chinese people, Liu Xiaoxiao rarely blames the gods or other people for his woes, putting everything down to fate. He often sighs and says, 'I have lousy luck.'

Back in Anlu, Liu Xiaoxiao finally comes to realise just how serious the catastrophe in Wuhan really is. He goes online, looking for answers. He had hoped to set his mind at ease but gradually he begins to wonder, *Is there something I should be doing to help?* 'I'm young and strong,' he says. 'Everyone is running away from the virus, but there are things that need to be done.'

The next morning, he posts a message on Weibo declaring he wants to return to Wuhan to be a volunteer. To demonstrate his determination, he adds a line fashionable at the time: 'No reward for me, regardless of the danger to my life.' The overconfident government has not made any preparations for ordinary citizens to participate in the aid program. Liu Xiaoxiao fills in an online form for volunteers, but when he telephones the Chinese Red Cross, the person who answers doesn't seem interested in his offer of help.

By 25 January, the virus has spread across the whole of China and has arrived in Thailand, Japan, the United States and many other countries. And on that day, the city of Anlu declares a lockdown. Every region in the country begins to ferret out travellers from Wuhan. Roads out of Hubei province are blocked off, many by excavating ditches across them. The province is now an island isolated in a vast ocean.

Liu Xiaoxiao reposts his Weibo message – 'No reward for me, regardless of the danger to my life' – and waits anxiously. The next day, things take a turn for the better. Three young women make contact with him online. They are nurses from a Wuhan hospital who need help to get back to Wuhan. Nurses and doctors have the highest level of laissez-passer, so Liu Xiaoxiao takes the opportunity to apply for a permit to leave Anlu and drive the three of them back to Wuhan on the freeway.

He had escaped from the city and now he has returned to fight a glorious battle.

Liu Xiaoxiao arrives in Wuhan on 27 January. He goes first to the Red Cross to volunteer, where he is assigned to answering the telephone.

After two days he begins to feel the work is 'boring' and 'unsatisfying'. He also feels guilty because at the Red Cross he is eating extremely well. Wuhan is short of food, medicine, beds – in fact, short of just about everything. Even the doctors battling to save lives on the front lines at the famous Wuhan Union Hospital only have instant noodles to stave off hunger. Yet at the Red Cross, there is more food than they can consume. 'Beautiful meal boxes, as many as you could eat,' says Liu Xiaoxiao. 'And then there was yoghurt and fruit, like apples and oranges, piled so high that no one there bothered to touch them. Breakfast was steamed buns, stuffed buns, eggs ... all in abundance.' He feels too uncomfortable and decides to leave. 'Wuhan was in a dire state. What's a young man like me doing gorging on fine food every day?'

Unlike in other countries, the Red Cross in China is not an independent charity; it's more like a subsidiary of the Chinese Communist Party. Senior administrators are mostly Party members. In recent decades it has been blighted by scandals, like officials embezzling donations to finance mistresses. On social media many call it the 'Black Cross Society', black for corrupt or evil. Now its vast funds sit idle. Urgently needed masks are diverted from frontline hospitals to private clinics that are not treating the virus.

Leaving the Red Cross behind, Liu Xiaoxiao joins a volunteer car pool to transport people who urgently need to travel. All public transport has ceased operation, and private cars are banned. Millions of people are confined to their homes, including doctors, nurses, pregnant women and people with critical illnesses.

Liu Xiaoxiao drives a cheap orange domestically made car, paying for the petrol himself, hurrying back and forth around the city, transporting people who need help. He's not paid a penny for his efforts, but he's happy.

He leaves home early in the morning and returns at night. It is very difficult to find a place to eat; all restaurants are closed. Sometimes people give him bread, crackers or eggs, and occasionally cooked food. At these times he is over the moon and takes snaps to share with his friends on social media, like a child showing off a new toy. 'Hot dry noodles are really tasty.' 'Soy sauce on rice, I can't ask for more.'

At the end of January, a restaurant in the Qiaokou district begins to hand out free meals, and Liu Xiaoxiao goes there several days in a row to 'freeload'. Standing by the side of the road with a lunch box in his hands, his heart brims with gratitude: 'How come there are so many kind people in the world?' He later posts a short video which he titles 'The food line brigade', showing a queue of at least one hundred cars driven by volunteers. 'It's not easy to get a meal,' he sighs. 'Just look at all those cars.' He mentions that some volunteers have come to blows over meal boxes.

Although Liu Xiaoxiao graduated from a top-tier university and is a teacher, he rarely thinks about what rights he deserves and is even less likely to fight for those rights. And yet, when his city encounters a disaster, he will step forward to help people in difficulty.

*

On 4 February, Liu Shiyu falls ill again, and the diagnosis is 'suspected viral infection'. It's a dangerous sign, prompting the nursing home to telephone Liu Xiaoxiao in Wuhan, instructing him to immediately take his father to a designated hospital for treatment.

The nursing home fees are cheap, but the food and service are cheap too. The air is often permeated with the rancid odour of sweat and urine. Liu Shiyu has been living there for a dozen-odd years and is frequently sick. But, says Liu Xiaoxiao, he's 'doing his best to get by'. The stroke affects Liu Shiyu's ability to talk and probably his cognitive functions too. He becomes obstinate and is extremely difficult to communicate with. In Liu Xiaoxiao's words, 'He's really inconsiderate.'

'How do I get Dad to a hospital? How?' Liu Xiaoxiao retorts. 'Everywhere is under lockdown. Can't leave Wuhan; can't leave Anlu.'

The nursing home is insistent: 'You must come, even if you have to walk.'

Liu Xiaoxiao is at a loss, shuffling from office to office asking for help, hoping to get a permit to leave Wuhan. He telephones his school, the Civil Affairs Department, the mayor's hotline, the Anlu Epidemic Command, the Wuhan Epidemic Command. Some ask for written documentation, which entails a whole new set of difficulties, going back and forth from one service to another. On 7 February, he finally receives a definitive answer: 'No.'

Liu Xiaoxiao says he can understand, because at that time Wuhan and the virus are synonymous. 'For other regions, people coming out of Wuhan represented a huge risk.'

Liu Xiaoxiao calls the 120 emergency hotline in Anlu in the hope they will deliver Liu Shiyu to the hospital. The operator says they are short-staffed.

Liu Xiaoxiao then calls the Anlu mayoral hotline, which replies disparagingly, 'You young people should be filial. Stop thinking you can just dump your parents on the government.' Liu Xiaoxiao defends himself by saying he does not want to shirk his responsibility. It never occurs to him that there could have been another response: 'Doesn't the government have an obligation to take care of citizens?'

There are laws requiring children to care for their parents. Those who shirk their responsibilities are not only branded unfilial, but may face criminal sanctions. Many old people who have fallen ill commit suicide because they don't want to burden their children.

On the evening of 7 February, as Wuhan residents roar with outrage over the death of Dr Li Wenliang, Liu Xiaoxiao issues a plea for help on Weibo: 'Is there a kind person somewhere who can take my father to the hospital?' There isn't. He reposts his message over and over, tagging it to government social media accounts, to the media in Beijing and Wuhan, to the rich and famous, but there is no reply.

Even at the nadir of despair, Liu Xiaoxiao never ceases to be understanding. 'Everyone has difficulties, but what can be done?' he posts on Weibo.

He tries to plead for help from the nursing home. The nursing home director says, 'You must come no matter what. You can't dump your father's problem onto me.' Liu Xiaoxiao begs the director. When begging achieves nothing, he argues. When arguing achieves nothing, he says he'll go to the media. He even says he'll report it to the governments of Wuhan city and Hubei province. The director responds: 'Even if you take the matter to a higher authority, in the end this nursing home will still have to handle it.'

Liu Xiaoxiao is enraged yet despondent. After a moment of sullen silence, he asks, 'If I pay? I'll pay any amount.'

It is a solution with an exorbitant price. Liu Xiaoxiao pays 10,000 RMB (A$2000) and the nursing home director helps him find a carer. On 9 February, the carer, Aunty Yang, takes Liu Shiyu to the hospital.

A few hours later Liu Xiaoxiao receives another phone call – Liu Shiyu is critically ill. Over the next week or two, the Anlu City Hospital fires off numerous 'critically ill' notifications. Liu Xiaoxiao is certain he is about to lose his father.

Then some different news arrives. Liu Shiyu has tested negative for the novel coronavirus, so the hospital is demanding Liu Xiaoxiao immediately take his father out of the hospital. He's astonished. 'You've been telling me he's critically ill so how can he be discharged?' The hospital responds, 'This is a special time: if he doesn't have the novel coronavirus, we don't have to treat him.'

Liu Xiaoxiao drags his feet for two days. On 19 February, the hospital presents an ultimatum: 'Liu Shiyu must leave the hospital.'

By now Liu Shiyu is extremely weak; he's almost unable to eat and can only sit up with difficulty. Worse, he has no place to go. Liu Xiaoxiao telephones the director of the nursing home to ask if his father can return. The director replies that, out of concern for cross infection, government regulations clearly stipulate that residents who leave nursing homes for treatment cannot return.

At 10 am on 20 February, a car sets out from the Anlu City Hospital. The passengers are Liu Shiyu and the carer, Aunty Yang. The car takes them to a remote place and stops. Here, Liu Shiyu and Aunty Yang are unceremoniously ejected in the middle of the road like unwanted merchandise.

Liu Xiaoxiao, stuck in Wuhan, says later that he felt helpless because he 'didn't know at whom to be angry'.

He has only one option left, an option that is every Chinese person's last – look for connections. He finds a former classmate who provides a telephone number. He then pleads with an official surnamed Wang, who turns out to be Liu Xiaoxiao's guardian angel. He gives Liu Xiaoxiao another telephone number, from which comes more telephone numbers, all of which Liu Xiaoxiao dials until he finally finds a place that will accept his father. It is a temporary bed in an Anlu restaurant that has closed down. In the following few days, Liu Shiyu, frail and without appetite, lives on a makeshift bed of wooden planks in the empty restaurant.

Liu Shiyu has a persistent low fever. The Anlu City Hospital says he doesn't have the coronavirus, but it doesn't say what he is suffering from or what treatment he needs. At dawn on 29 February, Liu Shiyu begins to vomit blood violently, splattering it over the bed and blankets. Aunty Yang takes a photograph and sends it to Liu Xiaoxiao, who springs into action. He follows the same routine, calling one number after another. At dawn the next day, Liu Xiaoxiao is finally able to send his father to another hospital in Anlu. The hospital provides some basic treatment and holds him for a few days.

On 8 March, Liu Shiyu is again forced out of the hospital; he must return to his wooden bed at the restaurant.

After a few more days, Liu Shiyu's condition worsens. He repeatedly vomits blood. At 2 am on 16 March, Liu Xiaoxiao sends a photo of Liu Shiyu to his friends on social media, showing his thin face, half-open eyes and the splatters of blood around his bed. Liu Xiaoxiao tells his friends that he himself is physically and mentally exhausted, and close to collapse. He can no longer let his father stay where he is in Anlu. He is determined to pool all his resources to bring his father to Wuhan.

Once again, Liu Xiaoxiao turns to Weibo and WeChat for assistance. He asks his fellow volunteers for help and he approaches radio and TV stations. Mr Wang, his guardian angel, comes to the rescue again, arranging a car to take Liu Shiyu to the edge of Wuhan. Later that day, Liu Xiaoxiao finally meets his father at the freeway entrance ramp. When he lifts his father, he is overcome by a wave of sadness. 'He was so much lighter than a few years earlier,' he says. 'There was no muscle on his legs, they were just stick-like bones.'

That afternoon, Liu Xiaoxiao embarks on yet another arduous journey: to find medical treatment for his father. He makes countless phone calls and seeks out dozens of people but is unable to find a single hospital bed. He spends hours dialling the emergency number of the Tongji Hospital. He finally gets through at 8 pm. A doctor tells him, 'Don't come. There are already too many people here and fights are about to break out.'

By that time, Liu Shiyu is close to death and unable to speak. Liu Xiaoxiao rushes his father to the Wuhan Union Hospital in the East-West Lake district. A doctor gives Liu Shiyu some basic treatment and arranges a

CT scan. The preliminary diagnosis excludes the novel coronavirus, but the hospital won't take him in.

Liu Xiaoxiao has no choice but to take his father out of the hospital into the cold of the night.

It has been a very long day. Utterly exhausted, Liu Xiaoxiao realises that he cannot look after his father and also handle all the complicated tasks at the hospital, like registering, lining up to pay the fees and taking his father to get all the tests. He can only turn to his friends for help. One of those friends is Xia Wenlun.

*

It's early January 2020. In a small city a thousand kilometres from Wuhan, Xia Wenlun feels abandoned. A few days earlier, his wife returned to her parents' house. She took their daughter but didn't invite Xia to join them.

Now in his forties, Xia Wenlun is a peculiar man. Although he has a university degree, he has had more than twenty jobs – factory worker, teacher, salesman, foot masseur. None has lasted very long.

When he was a masseur, he believed his foot massage technique could treat many diseases and even cure a woman's colon cancer. But he was the only one who believed it. His star sign is Capricorn, but according to China's Five Element physiognomy, his natal horoscope is 'Heavenly Fire'. He is convinced that he is on a mission.

'My horoscope is the same as Chairman Mao's,' he often boasts. Just before the epidemic started, Xia Wenlun saw an article online that 'smeared' the local Party secretary. Seeing it as an opportunity for himself, he printed the article and rushed to the city's Communist Party Committee compound, hoping to report to the Party secretary in person.

Xia doesn't think he was informing on someone. 'That was just providing information,' he says. He imagined the 'information' would be a ticket for him to enter China's market of power and money. 'No one in power is squeaky clean. If I help him, he will help me, then I will make it.' Unfortunately, he did not make it – the security guards didn't let him in. Xia argued back and forth with them briefly, then left, feeling dejected. But not for long. He has read the famous teachings of the ancient Chinese philosopher Mencius and understands that men destined for great things are meant to encounter all kinds of difficulties.

Xia spends Lunar New Year's Eve alone. He has rice and a plate of stir-fried Chinese broccoli. He also watches the dazzling New Year's Gala on CCTV. When the MCs gush about the unfolding disaster in Wuhan, Xia does not have the slightest concern. In fact, he is excited: something big is happening in China! For him, 'something big is happening' means an opportunity, though at the time he does not know how to seize the opportunity. He still has to wait for the right time. In Xia's words, 'My lucky moment had not arrived yet.'

Late on the evening of 7 February, Xia Wenlun is also heartbroken for Dr Li Wenliang. 'I even shed tears,' says Xia. He dials the Wuhan mayor's hotline and firmly demands the government name Dr Li a martyr. The girl who answers utters a few perfunctory words and hangs up. She probably can't understand Xia's thick accent or does not want to engage him in conversation. Xia is not surprised – he's used to setbacks and is good at thinking about failures positively. Two months later, when the Wuhan city government indeed names Li Wenliang a martyr, Xia is convinced he played a big role in this decision. 'See, I spoke to the Wuhan mayor about this a long time ago.' Xia is pleased, as pleased as if the spirit of a high-ranking official lived inside him.

The day of Xia Wenlun's 'lucky moment' finally arrives on 20 February; he hears that, 'according to the TV news, whoever goes to Wuhan to provide assistance will be named a martyr if he dies'. Xia is excited, thinking his time has come. He stuffs a few items of clothing into his backpack, takes his savings of 2500 RMB ($520), and sets off for Wuhan without saying goodbye to his wife and daughter.

Xia has no intention of becoming a martyr. 'I definitely won't die,' he says. 'Heaven will look after me.' He doesn't know what he can do in Wuhan, but he has great ambition and is confident of victory. 'I want to become a philanthropist. But a philanthropist has to have money. How to make money?' Eyes sparkling, he declares: 'I've thought it through. I must become famous first.'

He believes the journey to Wuhan will make him an online celebrity. 'When I return, the Party secretary and the mayor will come out to receive me,' he tells friends with confidence. No one believes him.

At the time, all transportation to Wuhan has stopped. Xia embarks on a long and tortuous route. He changes trains three times to arrive in Anhui province, which borders Hubei. In the following three days, he walks about 150 kilometres, from dawn to dusk. His feet are covered in blisters. 'It was piercingly painful.'

He walks through many villages and townships, meets many people and compiles many poems. Xia is a prolific poet. He's probably written tens of thousands of poems. The recurring subject is Mao Zedong, with whom he 'shares a natal horoscope'.

Every year on this day I commemorate you,
Grandpa Mao, in my heart.
Kneeling in front of your portrait,
I kowtow three times,
Paying respect to my hero Mao Zedong!

It is hard to arouse the interest of literary editors with poetry like this, but Xia never gives up. As he walks, blisters sting his feet but his poetic spirit is lively. He compiles poems about sunrise, about sunset, about tunnels and bridges, even about buns and instant noodles. Nothing can interrupt him when he talks about his poetry. 'I've written a poem,' he solemnly tells people. And if someone attempts to change the subject, he repeats loudly, 'I've written a poem – I've written a poem – I've written a poem.'

On 25 February, Xia arrives in Yingshan county in Hubei. Two volunteers pick him up. It's midnight by the time they arrive in Wuhan.

Watching the exhausted volunteers wolfing down instant noodles, Xia asks, 'How long have you been eating this?' Someone replies, 'We've been living on this for over a month.' Xia shakes his head: 'It's not nutritious and it's bad for health.' He looks at the people in the room. 'I don't want to eat this. Can someone find me some rice?'

Xia Wenlun joins a few volunteer organisations and participates in some of their group operations – unloading goods, transporting goods, delivering meals to homeless people. The volunteers are strangers to each other, but during those tense days they work together to help many overcome the hard times and they form a deep bond. They often refer to each other as 'comrades-in-arms'. They sincerely accept Xia Wenlun and at times share their true feelings with him.

But Xia is soon expelled from these organisations. 'Mr Xia is a strange man,' says a volunteer who knew him. 'He doesn't work hard and is picky about food and clothing. He makes odd remarks all the time and doesn't follow orders. He's really different from us.'

Xia has no idea what his colleagues say about him behind his back. 'I've done many good deeds,' he boasts, 'many, many good deeds.' On 2 March, he posts an article online titled 'A letter to a grandma in Wuhan', giving information about his background and mentioning 'our great Communist Party and government'. He describes how a speech by the new Party secretary in Wuhan 'moved me to tears'. He then describes in detail how he walked, 'despite the rain', to buy groceries for a Wuhan grandma. 'It was my honour to buy groceries for you. I bought carrots, white radish and cabbage. I also bought pork, soy sauce, vinegar, salt and the antiseptic liquid that you wanted, and shared with you fruit others had given me!'

This shopping excursion costs Xia over 100 RMB (A$21). The Wuhan granny attempts to pay him but Xia refuses to accept the money. The Wuhan granny's daughter and grandson want to pay him but, he writes, he refuses to accept their money too. Xia does not think he deserves gratitude. 'Your daughter and grandson thanked me, but I said no need. Please instead thank the central committee of the Communist Youth League.'

Xia insists he 'speaks with sincerity', but the sincerity may not be entirely genuine. He has nothing to do with the Communist Youth League. He is already in his forties, so he has not been a member for a long time, and he has never held a position in the organisation. It seems he hopes the article will attract the attention of the Communist Youth League, which will reward him for 'doing good deeds anonymously'. Sadly, his article does not attract much attention and his journey to fame remains a distant dream.

After posting the article, Xia 'picks up' a vagrant. The man, in his fifties, is destitute, cold and hungry after being stuck in Wuhan for many days. Xia brings the man back to his quarters, gives him food and even his own down jacket. Then, after displaying his kindness and generosity, he does something not so kind – he calls the police. 'Comrade police officer, there is a trapped person here ...'

The term 'trapped person' refers to a vagrant who has nowhere to go. During the lockdown in Wuhan, these people are affected badly. They cannot leave the city and there is nowhere to beg for food. In the bitterly cold winter of central China, they have to seek shelter under bridges, on construction sites, in abandoned buildings or even inside the Huanan Seafood Market. Government officials want them out of sight, so they are often chased away with batons, punches and ice-water guns, until March 2020, when the government finally shows a hint of compassion by allowing these people to take shelter indoors.

The police arrive at Xia's quarters in no time. They not only take away the vagrant but are also suspicious of Xia. He flees but is soon stopped by another group of police officers. 'I'm just a passer-by,' he tells the police, and refuses to show his ID. An officer steps forward to search Xia. 'You're violating the law while enforcing the law!' Xia yells. 'You are violating my human rights!'

At about midnight, Xia is locked up in a hotel together with dozens of 'trapped persons'. There are clean sheets and free food, but also strictly guarded doors with around-the-clock patrols. No one is allowed to leave without permission.

Xia stays there for three days. He has a few conversations with some trapped persons through the door but not a single conversation is pleasant. 'They were cursing,' Xia says. This makes him feel 'there is a lot of negative energy in that place'. 'No one could escape if there was a fire,' he says, with a lingering fear.

Xia decides to leave the place full of 'negative energy'. He smooth talks the guards: 'I'm a volunteer. I have work to do.' On 4 March, he solicits online a donation of over a dozen lunch boxes from a restaurant, then asks for help from other volunteers: 'Can anyone drive me to deliver some lunch boxes?'

A few seconds later, a volunteer by the name of 'East-West Lake Teacher Liu' responds. He picks up Xia from the hotel, then together they collect the lunch boxes and deliver them. In the following days, Xia partners with Teacher Liu many times to deliver meals to doctors, nurses and hungry volunteers. In those homeless nights, Xia camps in Teacher Liu's car. He's grateful and often praises Teacher Liu as a 'very radiant person'.

*

'I want to be someone who pursues the light,' Liu Xiaoxiao writes in a social media post. Still hard at work despite his father's state, he transports exhausted doctors and nurses, as well as canned food, instant noodles, frozen dumplings and medicines. He witnesses so much hardship – white-haired senior citizens lugging suitcases, pregnant women who deliver still-born babies, and people who prepare to walk dozens of kilometres home. He helps such people whenever he can, looking at it as a kind of redemption. 'I needed help, so I wanted to help others.'

Xia Wenlun is one of those in distress. The 2500 RMB he took with him when he left home is long gone and he has to rely on others to survive. He is now so scared of the police that he does not want to go out alone and needs to be chauffeured wherever he goes. After sleeping in Liu Xiaoxiao's car, he still cannot find a long-term place to stay. Every few days, he posts a message online: 'Please pick me up.' Some kind-hearted citizens in Wuhan host him but quickly become fed up with his fantastical babbling. Xia never thinks he is at fault. He always blames others for being 'too snobby' or 'having too much negative energy'.

In his days as a drifter, Xia never stops writing poetry. On his most productive days, he writes over a dozen poems like this one.

A resilient China!
Standing high in the Orient,
Bright as the Sun,
Even the United States looks up in admiration!

Xia Wenlun describes himself as a 'coordinator'. He doesn't know how to drive and doesn't have any resources. His biggest advantage is an abundance of spare time. He joins several WeChat groups in which some members need resources while others have resources to offer. Xia's job is to post messages in different groups: 'Who has masks?' or 'Who needs boxed meals?'

Liu Xiaoxiao finds it all quite amusing. 'Brother Xia is remarkable,' says Liu. 'He doesn't have much and can't do much, and yet he can be a volunteer.' Xia has 'coordinated' the delivery of masks, clothes and meal boxes worth over 10,000 RMB by the time Liu

Xiaoxiao posts his message pleading for help to manage his father's care.

Xia has joined a volunteer group called the China Traditional Chinese Medicine Practitioners Wuhan Medical Assistance Team, which has a rather poor reputation. The group consists of Taoist priests and Buddhist monks, as well as witch doctors and alchemists from all over the country. They wear peculiar costumes and behave strangely. Many of them don't have licences to practice but believe they possess magical techniques and superior skills. They risk their lives travelling to Wuhan during the novel coronavirus outbreak, hoping to participate in treating patients. However, no hospital is willing to accept their help. In the end, they dispense their magical cures to people who don't really need treatment.

Xia often helps them distribute their herbal medicines. According to his description, some of the medicines are gifts from god that can treat AIDS and leukaemia, as well as coughs and fevers. Convinced of their efficacy, Xia practises what he preaches, downing pack after pack of magical nostrums. This leads him to his life's mission: 'I've thought it through. My ideal now is' – and he articulates each of the following words separately – 'I. Want. To. Be. A. Miracle. Working. Doctor.'

Xia has no medical training, but for him that is no impediment. He believes in a mystical science called 'ethical therapy', which holds that all physiological ailments are connected to interpersonal relationships: 'What is the cause of headaches? Headaches are due to offending one's superiors, which means contradicting one's elders or the leaders.' By the same logic, lower back pain results from offending one's peers. Foot pain of course is due to offending subordinates or the younger generation.

As for Liu Shiyu's condition, Xia has no knowledge, but employing his theory he says, 'You should not let your father have an operation.' He tells Liu Xiaoxiao, 'You should give him Chinese herbal medicine.'

Liu Xiaoxiao does not follow his friend's advice. Early on 17 March, Liu Xiaoxiao and Xia carry Liu Shiyu back to the Wuhan Union Hospital. According to Xia, Liu Shiyu's hands are freezing cold and he is continuously coughing. He expels phlegm directly onto his mask. 'He went through over a dozen masks.'

They register him, and after a long wait a doctor comes. The doctor looks at the CT scan taken the previous day. 'Can't be treated,' he says bluntly. Liu Xiaoxiao is flabbergasted: 'Why can't such a big hospital treat him?' The doctor replies, 'Because your father has TB.'

Liu Xiaoxiao says he was 'very angry but could understand'. Tuberculosis is also an infectious disease and 'China has been traumatised by an infectious disease. Going to a hospital in that condition is a big deal.'

The doctor at the Wuhan Union Hospital recommends they go to a specialist lung hospital. It is 1 pm and the three of them have not had a chance to eat yet that day. But that isn't their biggest problem. Liu Xiaoxiao discovers that his father has wet his pants. Perhaps it happened because he is generally frail or has impaired bladder function, or perhaps after living in a nursing home for so long he does not ask for assistance and has become accustomed to urinating in bed or in his trousers.

This is a big test for Liu Xiaoxiao and he feels embarrassed because he always thinks of himself as a respectable person. 'How could I carry him into a hospital like that?'

Xia Wenlun is wearing three pairs of trousers. He takes off two pairs to give to Liu Shiyu. Liu Xiaoxiao is deeply moved. 'Up to this point in my life, to tell the truth, people have given money and words of support, but I've never seen anyone take off their trousers to help me. That was a first.'

With Xia's help, Liu Xiaoxiao takes Liu Shiyu to the lung hospital to undergo a battery of tests. Liu Xiaoxiao pays the various fees for the various tests, but in the end the hospital also refuses to admit Liu Shiyu. A kind old doctor tells them, 'The whole building is full of novel coronavirus patients. Your father probably has TB but that's not immediately fatal. The novel coronavirus is much more dangerous because it would be over in a few days if he were infected. Best take him home.'

Later, Liu Xiaoxiao learns that the doctor was not telling the truth, because on an upper floor in the hospital is a secret ward that admits patients with illnesses like Liu Shiyu's. As he carries his father out of the hospital, he thinks: 'Maybe it would be better if my father really had the novel coronavirus, because at least then he would be looked after.'

There is another pressing matter – Liu Xiaoxiao and his father now also need a place to live. Liu Xiaoxiao has a room in the dormitory of the school where he works, but the school will not permit Liu Shiyu to stay there because he has an infectious disease. 'A school is an important place, there can be no mishaps,' a school leader tells him, despite the fact that there is not a single soul in the school at that time. A relative has a spare room elsewhere in Wuhan, but all residential districts of Wuhan are under lockdown and Liu Xiaoxiao will never be able to sneak his father through the checkpoints. Liu Xiaoxiao tries hotels, but the answer is always the same: you can stay, but your father can't.

It is the most beautiful season in Wuhan and the cherry trees are blossoming without a single tourist in sight. Liu Xiaoxiao drives his father from place to place, to no avail, while making phone calls and repeating his story to all sorts of people. But he just can't find a place for them to stay.

Behind him, the shrunken Liu Shiyu, who hasn't eaten a grain of rice for an entire day, is crumpled in the back seat croaking, 'Let's go, let's go.'

Liu Xiaoxiao drives from East-West Lake to Baishazhou, then from Baishazhou to Zhong Family Village, and then from Zhong Family Village back again. A crisp spring breeze carries wave after wave of pink and white cherry blossom petals to the ground. Liu Xiaoxiao stops his car to frantically type mistake-riddled messages to his social media friends. He expresses empathy for others – the hospitals, the residential areas, the hotels and the school that shut him out. He doesn't blame them because they are following regulations. He then asks in desperation: is it possible for the entire population of Wuhan to help me call the mayor's hotline?

Sitting behind him, the incontinent, unfed, gravely ill old man continues to croak, 'Let's go, let's go.'

In the last few minutes of that long day, the law-abiding Liu Xiaoxiao finally violates a rule. He takes his father to the school, furtively carries him up to the seventh floor and gently places him on his own bed. He knows that as soon as he is discovered he will be in a lot of trouble, but he can't worry about that. 'My father hadn't eaten all day and if he didn't get a good night's sleep, would he survive?'

Liu Xiaoxiao himself is only sleeping two or three hours a night. 'I felt I had expended all my fuel.' And he is fearful of getting sick. 'That would be the end.'

The next day at noon, he carries his father down to his car. Before he starts the car, he sees his award certificate and its legend: 'Thank you for guarding the world.' Some days earlier, a company presented him with the award for helping several hundred people. It was the same day Vice Premier Sun Chunlan led a contingent of officials to a Wuhan residential compound where the occupants, enraged by the government's propaganda, shouted, 'Fake, fake, it's all fake.'

Looking at the certificate, Liu Xiaoxiao bursts into tears. Because his father is in the car, he cries silently, hands on the steering wheel, tears streaming down his cheeks. 'I'm thanked for guarding the world, but what have I really guarded?' he asks himself. 'My father is in this sorry state and there's nothing I can do.'

In Liu Xiaoxiao's view, all this – poverty, sickness, death, being humiliated and despised – is linked to fate. *Is it possible all the troubles in this life*, he begins to think, *are because I did bad things in a previous life and owe a huge debt to fate?* It's Chinese Buddhist teaching, but Liu Xiaoxiao is not a Buddhist. He says he'd 'prefer to believe in communism'.

His fate soon takes another turn. An official permits his father to temporarily live in the school dormitory – by pretending he is unaware of the situation. Liu Xiaoxiao is deeply grateful because now they won't need to camp outdoors. Several days later, a journalist helps him contact another hospital. Liu Xiaoxiao takes his father there and is able to register him. After several examinations, the cause of his father's illness is diagnosed: in addition to TB, there is serious bleeding in the lungs. The doctor puts together a treatment plan.

On 26 March, Liu Xiaoxiao pays 20,000 RMB (A$4100) in advance for an operation – almost all of his savings. The hospital also requires that he buy a new set of PPE, as well as straws, toilet paper and mineral water, all necessary for the operation. Finally, Liu Xiaoxiao breathes a sigh of relief as he watches his father get rolled into the operating theatre.

Two days later, Liu Xiaoxiao receives the bill. The total outstanding for the operation and the various other expenses is over 40,000 RMB. Liu Xiaoxiao is frantic. Chinese hospitals are not known for compassion. Medical fees must be paid in advance, and if payment for continuing treatment is not made, hospitals take extreme measures, like holding back medicines or initiating legal action.

Liu Xiaoxiao panics for two days but cannot think of anything better than making a public appeal for assistance.

He sets up a Douyin account (the Chinese version of TikTok) and posts a short video every day, mostly about food. On 28 March it is black rice porridge, on 29 March it is egg broth, on 30 March, soft noodles.

In the videos, Liu Xiaoxiao wears a black face mask as he ladles spoonful after spoonful into Liu Shiyu's mouth. There is background music as he explains his story.

This 'Diary of saving my father' attracts a lot of attention. People not only express their good wishes, they also loosen their purses to help. By 8 April, when the lockdown on Wuhan is lifted, over 1500 ordinary people have made donations to a total exceeding 100,000 RMB (A$20,000).

On 10 April, after paying off all the medical bills, Liu takes his father home to their little dormitory room on the seventh floor. He prepares three meals a day, bathes his father, and cleans up his vomit and excreta. He also manages to fit in teaching his students online. The Wuhan lockdown is over; the volunteer car pool is disbanded. Liu Xiaoxiao receives several medals and award certificates proving that in a catastrophe he heroically 'guarded the world'.

At 5 am on 11 April, he drives some volunteers to a place called Caitian to see off the People's Liberation Army personnel who had been transferred to Wuhan to help. He stands at the side of the road with his friends, bowing in respect as each military truck drives by, shouting, 'Thanks to the soldiers of the people, we are all one family.'

Liu Shiyu will die at 8 pm on the eighth day of the eighth month of 2020. According to Chinese superstition, it is an auspicious time – there are three eights. The number eight sounds like the word for prosperity. Perhaps the three eights preordain that in Liu Shiyu's next life he will be rich, and not live in poverty, isolation, hardship and grime. Liu Xiaoxiao posts a message to his WeChat contacts, announcing his father's death. 'My father didn't make it through to the end of 2020,' he writes. 'I brought him to Wuhan on 16 March this year. I was a filial son in the last five months of his life. It's almost a happy ending.'

Liu Xiaoxiao arranges his father's cremation. Two days later, he buries the ashes in a cemetery. The funeral is simple – no memorial speech, not many tears or much grief. Like tens of thousands of nameless people who die during the pandemic, Liu Shiyu's life and death are like a blade of grass whirled up by the wind, landing eventually on the ground, silently turning into dirt.

With tears streaming down his face, Liu Xiaoxiao writes on WeChat, 'Father, have a safe journey. This is the last send-off. You looked after me for eighteen years and I looked after you for sixteen years. This is the end of us as father and son. Goodbye.'

*

After the lockdown is lifted, Xia Wenlun stays in Wuhan for two months more. He has no long-term abode, no job and no money. One day, he admits he doesn't have

10 RMB on him. 'Even a dog has to eat to survive,' he laments. More kind-hearted people give him some food, a boxed meal or a pack of instant noodles. Sometimes people still take him in for a day or two. At such times Xia says, 'Grateful for the encounter.'

'Grateful for the encounter. It had been a week and I finally took a hot shower. A sister who I had never met before brought me to her home. I had warm food and a shower head to toe!'

Perhaps because Xia has consumed too much dubious herbal medicine, his liver, lungs and blood vessels all have problems. 'I am not feeling well but I want to live, live healthily,' he writes to WeChat friends. 'Who can help me? Who can save me?'

He goes to various hospitals, hoping to find a carer's job. In those two months, he looks after many patients. One is a ninety-three-year-old man, another a cancer patient called Yaoyao. Xia looks after her for twenty-one days and often treats her using his 'miracle massage' technique. 'I performed emergency treatment on her at least forty times.' But in the end, Yaoyao dies. The news devastates Xia. He sheds many tears and writes many poems.

Xia does his best to help others. He often initiates donations for strangers in his WeChat groups, helping them collect food, medicine, medical equipment and, of course, money. This plague-stricken city never disappoints him. Every plea for help and call for donations receives responses. 'Grateful for the encounter. A city full of kind people,' he sighs.

Xia finally returns to his home hundreds of kilometres away in the middle of June. He doesn't become an online celebrity or a miracle-working doctor. The mayor and Party secretary of the city don't receive him either. Yet Xia – the dreamer, the believer in every belief, the volunteer, the wandering poet – does not return empty-handed. He writes:

If one day
You no longer yearn for success,
Just do something.
If one day
You no longer yearn for love,
Just follow love.
No longer yearn for success,
Just work for it,
That is the real beginning.

When Xia returns to his old life, everything is the same. He has no job, no money, and no one likes him. His wife repeatedly asks for a divorce, but he never agrees. Xia will probably never become as successful as he is in his fantasies, but he never ceases to burn with warmth for the world.

Xia often thinks about his days in Wuhan. At the moment when tens of thousands of people were living in horror, he entered the sealed city alone. He was rejected, chased away, treated as a burden or a trouble, yet he did his best to help many, like a beggar sharing food with an even hungrier beggar. As 2020 draws to an end, he remembers fondly the mountain ranges and open fields along the Yangtze River, the deserted city with its brilliant lights, and the cherry blossoms tossed about in the spring showers that felt like a lover's hand.

I do not write a will
Because I don't yet want to die
I silently cry
For the homeless people on the street, I silently cry
I want to be a beam of light
To light up the darkness.

5.

My soul is singing

Zhang Zhan will never forget the scene that confronted her when she dragged her dilapidated wheelie suitcase out of the Hankou Railway Station.

'It was like Chernobyl,' says Zhang Zhan. 'The whole city was deserted. Not a single person in sight. No vehicles. The skyscrapers looked like giant monsters silently observing me. It felt like all that was left on earth was just me and those monsters. I've never seen anything like that before.'

It was the first day of February, the tenth day of Wuhan's lockdown. According to unreliable official statistics, Wuhan already had more than four thousand cases of the novel coronavirus and 224 had died. Zhang Zhan never believes such statistics and in fact is deeply suspicious of every single word the government utters. It is one reason she travelled to Wuhan – she wants to expose the lies.

Before 2016, Zhang Zhan lived a comfortable and respectable life. She had legal residency in Shanghai. She is a lawyer with a master's degree, and earned a good income as an investment officer at a large stockbroking firm. 'I was a member of the petty bourgeoisie with vested interests,' she says with remorse, like a criminal recalling her own crimes.

In May 2016, the stockbrokers fired Zhang Zhan. 'The boss wanted me to falsify accounts and I refused.' Soon after that, her lawyer's accreditation was revoked because she publicly opposed the newly amended Lawyers Law of the People's Republic of China.

Four years later, Zhang Zhan calmly speaks of these changes as if discussing food or the weather. But at the time they were a huge blow, the biggest setback she had experienced. They changed her life, but also changed her outlook on the country and the regime.

Zhang Zhan did not look for another job because she believes China's financial industry is utterly corrupt. 'False accounting and lies everywhere. How can that be called a financial industry?' she asks. 'A real financial industry creates wealth for the country's citizens, but in China the politically powerful harvest the wealth through "white-gloved" proxies.' She began to post articles online criticising China's finance industry and financial policies, and companies like Huawei and ZTE. 'Huawei and ZTE are ridiculous. How can they be the backbone of China? They're just pilferage workshops.'

The Chinese government did not appreciate her opinions. Soon, her articles were deleted, one after another, and so was her social media account. She became more impassioned by the day. She sharply criticised the government's excessive issue of currency, which she called a 'spigot of cheating'. In June 2018, she lamented that if the central bank continued to open the spigot, she would be forced to join the ranks of the starving. Soon after that, in an angry and dispirited moment, she even said she'd go to Beijing to blow up the Gate of Heavenly Peace. At the time she never expected her words would bring her so much trouble.

The Gate of Heavenly Peace is the ancient portal to China's imperial city, the symbol of the imperial family's authority and majesty. China's communist leaders are quite partial to this enormous fifteenth-century city gate tower. Every chairman of the Communist Party from Mao Zedong to Xi Jinping has stood on the ramparts to inspect military parades or officiate over ceremonial events. In some ways, the Gate of Heavenly Peace is the embodiment of the Communist Party.

Late one night in September 2018, there was a knock on the door. Zhang Zhan opened the door and several police officers pushed their way in. They searched her apartment thoroughly, looking for explosives. None were found and neither were any tools that might be used for a criminal purpose. She was so frightened and confused that she forgot to ask to see the search warrant.

After the search, the police forced her to move out of her Shanghai neighbourhood. 'They herded me to Huinan Town,' says Zhang Zhan, as if she were livestock. Such punishments have no basis in law, but Zhang Zhan was so fed up with the constant harassment that she took all her belongings and moved to Huinan Town, a remote residential area south-east of Shanghai. It meant she had to forsake her previous comfortable life and embark on her battle with the regime.

One day in early March 2019, Zhang Zhan walked into the Huinan subway station and held up a banner upon which she'd written: 'Down with the Communist Party, End Socialism'.

It was a very dangerous act. Zhang Zhan was afraid, so afraid she doesn't remember how long she stood there. 'A few dozen seconds, maybe more than one minute, anyway no more than five minutes.' She then rushed home. The police were already there, waiting for her.

She was taken to a detention centre and locked up for more than forty days. To investigate the origins of her criminality, the police said she would undergo a psychiatric evaluation. Zhang Zhan immediately thought of Dong Yaoqiong, the young girl known as the 'Ink Girl'. Dong Yaoqiong splashed ink on a portrait of Xi Jinping on a street in Shanghai while shouting, 'I oppose the dictatorial tyranny of Xi Jinping.' She was quickly sent to a psychiatric hospital, where she was held for almost a year. Incarcerating mentally sound people in psychiatric hospitals is an increasingly common tactic used by the Chinese government against 'petitioners' and dissidents.

The thought made Zhang Zhan shudder. 'I was fearful of being turned into a psychiatric case,' she says. 'That would be the biggest humiliation.'

Zhang Zhan vehemently resisted a psychiatric evaluation. The detention centre tried a more conciliatory approach. Two plain-clothed officers were dispatched to have a chat with her. She was unaware they were forensic investigators. She revealed her true feelings and talked about the significance of sin in Christianity. 'I have sinned, we all have sinned,' she explained. The forensic investigators probably misunderstood what she meant, but nonetheless certified that Zhang Zhan 'is able to take criminal responsibility', meaning that she was aware of and in control of her actions and not a psychiatric case.

The assessment was very important to Zhang Zhan. In the coming years, as she progressed further down her chosen path, every time she was abused and humiliated, when the pain became unbearable, she would often fall into deep self-doubt and ask herself, *What is this for? Am I crazy?* Then she remembered the psychiatric evaluation and used it to encourage herself. *No, I'm not a psychiatric case. Everything I have done, ought to have been done.*

After forty days, Zhang Zhan was released from the detention centre. But her life did not change for the better. As she saw it, she merely moved from a small prison to a larger one.

Secret police kept her under constant surveillance. They followed her. Her family was harassed, as were her classmates, friends and teachers. The secret police went to Xi'an and Chengdu to find anyone who had ever been in contact with her and investigated everything about her. They vilified her, claiming she had a psychiatric illness or that she took black money from foreigners. 'It's painful too when close friends say I am a lunatic,' says Zhang Zhan.

Sometimes they confronted her directly to humiliate and rebuke her, calling her verminous: 'You can't care for your parents, still you make them worry about you.' Sometimes the secret police flaunted their omniscience and omnipotence. 'Hey. We know where you've been and who you've seen, and we know what you've done.' This made Zhang Zhan anxious. 'Sometimes it felt like they were in step with my brain, that they knew what I was thinking.'

But she was not cowed. On 8 September 2019, she walked down Shanghai's bustling Nanjing East Road carrying a large blue umbrella on which was written: 'End Socialism, Down with the Communist Party'. She walked down the road for twenty minutes hoping people would notice, but from beginning to end not a single person said a word to her. That's Shanghai, the richest city in China, where people are too busy making money.

The next day, Zhang Zhan was arrested again, charged with 'disturbing public order'. The charge was later amended to 'picking quarrels and provoking trouble'. These two criminal offences under Chinese law are used for all acts that displease the government – street brawls, making a racket, graffiti, petitioning, expressing opinions on social media. Zhang Zhan's 'crimes' are much more serious, but the government will not admit she is a political prisoner. Just two months later, the Chinese Ambassador to London Liu Xiaoming tells the BBC that China has no political prisoners. Therefore, Zhang Zhan is only qualified to be a picker of quarrels and a provoker of trouble.

The police again took Zhang Zhan to a detention centre and locked her in a room with petitioners, drug users and prostitutes. It gave Zhang Zhan a deeper insight into the nature of China's legal system. 'I used to think that prisons were for locking up criminals,' she says, 'but after being on the inside I discovered that these people are all in for trivial matters – one month for prostitution, one month for playing mahjongg. A little old lady who collects rubbish with a trishaw was also locked up for a month. They are the marginalised and disadvantaged. Where are all the real criminals?'

Perhaps out of a desire to arouse a spirit of resistance in the other inmates, Zhang Zhan delivered speeches in her prison cell. The first day of October 2019 was the communist regime's seventieth-anniversary celebration. While Xi Jinping presided over the huge military parade in Beijing at Tiananmen Square, showing off his military might to the world, Zhang Zhan was making a 'reactionary speech' in a crowded Shanghai prison cell. Standing inside the iron door, she shouted to the free air outside: 'We have the right to not love this country!'

On another occasion, during the Sino–US trade negotiations in November 2019, the Chinese government held a grand trade expo in Shanghai at which Xi Jinping delivered a speech, promising the VIPs from around the world that China would further open up, that 'China will reach out with open arms'. Zhang Zhan's prison cell was overflowing with more and more petty offenders, and she became angrier and angrier. From her cell, she loudly criticised China's judicial system and described the police as 'evil accomplices': 'They intensify China's darkness.' She denounced the flashy pageant. 'The government squandered so much money. Why not use it to solve the basic needs of the people?'

Zhang Zhan's speeches infuriated the leadership of the detention centre. A very loud prison guard with the intimidating habit of wearing a belt on the outside of her tunic (Zhang Zhan thought she closely resembled

Chairman Mao) angrily rebuked Zhang Zhan for wanting to 'rebel'. 'The Communist Party raised you,' she boomed, 'so show a bit of gratitude.'

Zhang Zhan was unyielding. 'My parents raised me. What's that got to do with the Communist Party?'

'Chairman Mao' replied with her master blow, demanding Zhang Zhan admit the error of her ways. 'If you don't, it's solitary confinement.'

Zhang Zhan raised her head high. 'I'm not wrong!'

Those three words cost Zhang Zhan seven days in solitary. It may have been more than seven days because she lost her sense of time. She was locked in a windowless room with four iron hoops on the floor to which her hands and feet were shackled, preventing her from turning over. She lay on the cold, damp floor, from where she had to do all her daily tasks – eat, drink, urinate, defecate.

When Zhang Zhan later recounts her humiliations to her friends, she shows not the slightest hint of anger or sorrow. She just says softly, 'It was truly a torment.' Zhang Zhan does not like to describe her own travails. She speaks fluent English yet apologises for her inelegant writing. She is excessively polite, like a Japanese person, and it is her manner to try in every situation to maintain a graceful demeanour. When talking with strangers she often says, 'Excuse me for bothering you.'

At the very moment that honoured guests from around the world are clinking glasses in the spectacular banquet hall for the trade expo in Shanghai, Zhang Zhan is locked in a dark room, lying in her own excrement. That night she sees a gaggle of little devils flying in front of her face. She thinks she is about to die, but at that same moment she hears the sound of singing, carefree and without worries, like the sound of heaven, coming from within her own body. Listening to the singing she suddenly feels joyful and blessed. 'I believe people have souls,' she says. 'That was my soul singing.'

When solitary confinement ended, Zhang Zhan experienced serious medical problems and occasionally suffered incontinence. The seven days shackled in complete darkness left her feeble and virtually unable to move about without support from others.

The detention centre again raised the spectre of a psychiatric evaluation. Zhang Zhan vehemently refused. 'I went on hunger strike twice, once for three days and once for two and a half days.' Perhaps 'Chairman Mao' admired Zhang Zhan's courage because she dropped the idea of the evaluation. But they forced her to sign a document certifying she was healthy and had not been tortured or mistreated.

Soon after the grand trade expo concluded, Zhang Zhan's brother picked her up from the detention centre and took her back to his home; she couldn't return to her own Shanghai residence, because while she was away the police had 'assisted' the surrender of her rental property and disposed of her personal items.

Zhang Zhan spent most of her time lying in bed. She never considered hospital treatment. 'Hospitalisation costs money and I haven't worked for quite a few years.'

One morning at breakfast, Zhang Zhan's brother asked her to leave Shanghai. She refused and the two of them began to argue back and forth, until he angrily slapped her face.

Zhang Zhan says she can understand that slap, explaining haltingly, 'The police gave him so much pressure ... It was hard for him ... He had always looked after me ... I'm not a good sister.' Even so, that slap was deeply hurtful for Zhang Zhan, and from that day on she did not speak with her brother again. She dragged her weakened body out of her brother's home, although she had nowhere to go.

In China, people like Zhang Zhan are often very lonely. Her brother never understood why Zhang Zhan was doing what she has been doing – which brought not only the catastrophe of incarceration to her, but also big trouble to her entire family. Her parents disapproved of her; her middle-class friends looked down on her. Even her lover felt she was too radical and left her.

A priest from an underground church heard about her plight and took her in for a few days. Her health began to improve, but it wasn't long before the police ordered the church to send her on her way. It was an order that couldn't be ignored, so Zhang Zhan had to move again. Later, the police closed down the church, forcing several hundred of the faithful out into the freezing streets. Zhang Zhan feels terribly guilty for involving the church, but in the eyes of the priest she needn't have. 'Even without Zhang Zhan, we would still be harassed.'

*

In January 2020, Zhang Zhan spends Lunar New Year's Eve alone in a small rented room. She watches the TV news reports about the Wuhan pneumonia and feels she should go there to see for herself. 'Such a severe disaster, so many people suffering pitifully,' she says. 'That place definitely needs help.'

Shanghai is in a high state of anxiety, which provides Zhang Zhan a degree of freedom because the secret police are terrified. She purchases a train ticket to Chongqing. After she's been sitting on the train for about five hours, the secret police learn of her movements. They ask her mother to call Zhang Zhan to find out why she is going to Chongqing. Zhang Zhan replies: 'I'm not going to Chongqing, I'm already in Wuhan.'

Her mother asks: 'What will you do in Wuhan?' Zhang Zhan doesn't answer. She smiles and hangs up, saying to herself, 'I've finally escaped'.

As the train enters Wuhan station, Zhang Zhan drags her suitcase to the carriage door. A train conductor asks, 'You're getting off?' Zhang Zhan nods.

'Wuhan is very dangerous now.'

'I know.'

The door opens, and Zhang Zhan disembarks. At thirty-seven, Zhang Zhan has no partner, no work, no money, and no idea what she will do in Wuhan. Still, she has come. It is early afternoon in central China. There is a slight chill in the breeze as Zhang Zhan faces the bright daylight and steps into the huge, desolate city.

Later, journalists ask why she went to Wuhan. Her answers vary. Sometimes she says she was spreading the gospel. At other times, she says she was comforting the sick.

Neither are her true purpose.

In the 104 days she spends in Wuhan, she rarely encounters novel coronavirus patients and only spreads the gospels once. In a residential district one day at the end of February, she holds several dozen folded sheets of paper on which are printed, 'Reasons to believe in Jesus – apart from Him, there is no salvation.' She hands out the leaflets but they don't arouse any religious fervour; instead, the residents treat her coldly, some with obvious hatred in their eyes. Zhang Zhan does not understand why they hate her, but from that point on she doesn't try to spread the gospel again.

She stays in a cheap hotel, eats the simplest food and goes to many dangerous places. 'I was hurrying around the city bumping about like a headless fly,' says Zhang Zhan. 'I often asked myself, what am I doing?'

The Chinese government has been boasting that the newly constructed Huoshenshan Hospital is a glorious victory in the epidemic-prevention battle, an embodiment of the superiority of the system, evidence of the Communist Party's wisdom. On 4 February, Zhang Zhan decides to visit the famous hospital. She rides a bicycle for five hours, manages to pass an army checkpoint, and sneaks in through a small gap in the fence.

'It was a huge construction site,' says Zhang Zhan. 'Only a small section had been completed, where a plaque saying "Intensive Care Ward" was hanging. Elsewhere, building materials like rebars and bags of concrete were stacked high. Construction completed? There were construction workers chatting and smoking. Almost none had personal protection equipment. It was heartbreaking to see their filthy face masks.'

Zhang Zhan posts what she witnessed on social media, expecting it to demolish the lies of official media, but her posts don't attract much attention. At that time, the government has already told so many lies, bigger lies than those Zhang Zhan uncovers. In the end, the truth she uncovers with such difficulty is drowned out by the ear-piercing noise created by the country's propaganda machinery.

She visits several other hospitals and even walks into the fever wards. She finds no information of interest and rarely manages to talk to patients. To this day, some 80,000 people have been treated for the coronavirus in Wuhan, but few are willing to tell their stories.

On 7 February, Zhang Zhan posts a four-minute talk on YouTube to mourn the passing of Dr Li Wenliang. She speaks up for the importance of freedom of speech: 'Without freedom of speech, every one of us is Li Wenliang.' Perhaps because she has not done enough preparatory work, her talk is a bit incoherent; when discussing constitutional rights, she looks as if she is about to cry.

In the four-minute talk, Zhang Zhan's soft voice, somewhat melancholic, is also expressing her rage.

Her WeChat account is cancelled that day. She applies for another but within two hours the new account is also cancelled. The secret police in Shanghai instruct her mother to tell her that if she keeps on making trouble, she will be held in isolation again. Zhang Zhan feels hurt. 'Why are you siding with the police?' she asks her mother. Then she says, stony-hearted, 'You should all go on and live well, just let me die by myself.'

The YouTube talk brings her many supporters. Some praise her courage, some say she has a nice voice, and some are concerned, reminding her that her path is one of no return.

Zhang Zhan is certain that everything she has done is god's will, but the support of people is hugely important, perhaps even more important. Many people admire her for heroically going towards danger while everyone else is trying to flee. They donate money to her, some 36,000 RMB (A$7300) from early February to the end of March. After arriving in Wuhan with hardly a penny to her name, the donations encourage her, enabling her to persevere in difficult circumstances. However, she soon decides not to accept any more donations because they would lead to laziness. 'I was not after money,' says Zhang Zhan. 'I will keep pushing forward until they either arrest me or I die of starvation.'

When Zhang Zhan mentions starving to death, it is not merely a rhetorical flourish. She recalls that after Wuhan was locked down there really was a period of starvation for some. Each day she goes out early in the morning and returns late at night, often only eating one meal a day. 'When I couldn't find anything to eat, I had to go hungry.'

It is the same for finding a place to stay. Most hotels are closed or only accept out-of-town medical personnel. Zhang Zhan does not have much choice other than cheap family hostels. However, because they are of poor quality, too costly or out of the way, she is often dragging her suitcase from one location to another. Public transport is suspended, so she mostly walks. Occasionally, she finds an illegal motorcycle taxi. She feels sympathy for the city's poorest people, who risk their lives to get customers. When she talks with them, she comes to understand the difficulties the pandemic and the reckless lockdown inflicts on such people. On 4 or 5 February, she meets a motorcycle taxi driver. His vehicle is broken-down, his clothes are wretched; even his face mask is tattered, as if he'd been wearing it for many days. Feeling sick at heart, Zhang Zhan gives him a brand-new one. 'These people in the lowest level of society are truly pitiful,' she sighs.

Like Fang Bin, Chen Qiushi, Li Zehua, Fang Fang and others, Zhang Zhan is called a 'citizen journalist'. This appellation is more complex than the words suggest. Citizen journalist implies true reporting, standing with the people, and at the same time a kind of quiet rebellion. During Wuhan's lockdown, information too was locked down; people could only watch the government bragging, unable to learn how people were actually coping in Wuhan. This is why Fang Fang's daily diary posts were so well-received. Fang Bin's reports went one step further – he filmed chaotic hospital scenes of exhausted doctors and rows of corpses. Such scenes are never shown on government TV stations.

On 7 February, Fang Bin, already under house arrest, posts his own moving talk, shedding tears over the death of Dr Li Wenliang. In an act of extraordinary courage, he declares the Communist Party to be an evil cult: 'This pandemic is not just a natural disaster, it is also a man-made disaster. The Chinese communist tyranny is the systemic reason for this pandemic. It is their stupidity that enabled the epidemic to spread all over China and then the whole world.' He holds his hands high and shouts: 'People of China, fear not. Unite to resist tyranny!'

Zhang Zhan finds Fang Bin's talk inspirational, but at the same time she feels guilty because she did not stand up to support him soon enough. She says she was 'very nervous', then frankly admits, 'This is a mistake I made.'

In the following days, Zhang Zhan resists the authorities more fiercely, frequently clashing with the police. Perhaps she is thinking of Fang Bin and the mistake that cannot be considered a mistake.

On 9 February, Fang Bin could no longer be contacted. He hasn't been heard from since.

*

On 10 February, when Wuhan starts locking down neighbourhoods, Zhang Zhan is staying in a family hostel near the Wuchang train station. The neighbourhood committee issues a pass document stipulating that each family can send out one person once every three days. Zhang Zhan ignores the rules and continues to leave early and return late. She goes to the Wuchang morgue, a cabin hospital and the Wuhan Institute of Virology, trying to find a way in to the P4 laboratory that is making the whole world feel ill at ease. But she still comes up empty-handed.

Four days later, there is another knock on her door.

As she opens the door, Zhang Zhan feels as if she has walked onto a Hollywood sci-fi movie set. Three visitors from the distant future stand in front of her. They wear white protective clothing, masks and goggles. They measure her temperature and question her about her personal details and movements. Then they tell her: 'A neighbour has reported you, so now you'll have to stay in isolation for fourteen days. Quickly go and buy supplies.'

Zhang Zhan cannot endure this treatment, so the next day she drags her suitcase out of that district and moves to a small hotel on Old Railway Station Road. The residential neighbourhood lockdown escalates; no one can enter or leave the district. The entrances are guarded. All daily necessities – grain, vegetables, medicines – must be purchased online or through the neighbourhood committee.

Zhang Zhan, like all Wuhan inhabitants, is stranded inside a residential neighbourhood. She writes several essays and posts a lot of videos vehemently criticising the 'violent isolation', suggesting the government is using epidemic prevention as an excuse to enslave the people, a kind of a 'fascist management method'. Then, naturally, her WeChat accounts disappear, one after another, for 'suspicion of spreading malicious rumours'.

Zhang Zhan searches everywhere and finally discovers a small path to sneak out of the neighbourhood. She usually sets out late at night, squeezing out through a small gap in a remote corner. She again goes to several hospitals and the Wuhan Institute of Virology. She visits the Huanan Seafood Market but is unable to uncover any information about the virus there and only sees people destroying goods, which she says is 'unscientific' – she suspects the government is destroying evidence. At midnight on 18 February, Zhang Zhan rides a bicycle to the Wuhan crematorium, hoping to find out the number of deceased. She waits outside the crematorium for over an hour, cold and hungry. She does not see the expected convoy of vehicles transporting corpses. All she hears is the eerie din of late-night cremations.

This is Zhang Zhan's period of instant soup noodles and hot dry noodles. In one month, she eats five catties (2.5 kilos) of dry noodles and two cases of instant noodles. She does not buy vegetables from the neighbourhood group purchases because the prices are exorbitant. She has seen the 'relief vegetables' distributed during the lockdown, which the official media report as an expression of Party and government concern for the people. Zhang Zhan is disdainful: 'When I saw those vegetable packs, I wanted to cry. Two garlic sprouts, a rotten winter melon, mouldy bell peppers – that's what they called a relief pack.'

Like all Wuhan residents in those difficult days, Zhang Zhan experiences pain and sorrow. She comes across many desperate people. One day she sees an out-of-towner at the entrance to a residential district. Penniless, with nowhere to go, he is pleading for help from passers-by. Zhang Zhan gives him 100 RMB (A$21), but she is deeply worried for him. 'I don't know where he went or what became of him.'

An eighty-year-old man living alone can't get around and does not know how to use a smartphone to pay for food. In more than forty days of lockdown, he has only eaten relief vegetables twice. Zhang Zhan frequently visits him, her heart full of sympathy. 'Poor old man. If it weren't for neighbours giving him food,' she sighs, 'he would not have survived.'

March 7 is the forty-fourth day of Wuhan's lockdown. Some call it 'China's Black Thanksgiving'. According to the government, on that day Wuhan has had close to 50,000 novel coronavirus cases and 2370 deaths. Several million people are suffering the daily indignities of material shortages and feelings of dejection. The new Wuhan Party secretary, Wang Zhonglin, appears on the TV news. He wears a blue face mask and gesticulates as he flatters Xi Jinping for 'personally deploying and personally commanding'. He announces that the Wuhan government has plans to educate the people in how to express their gratitude, to 'thank the Communist Party Secretary General, thank the Communist Party, obey the Communist Party, follow the Communist Party to create forceful positive energy'.

Wang Zhonglin's toadying enrages the public. With her camera on, Zhang Zhan asks people in her residential district if they feel grateful. A middle-aged man tactfully responds, 'If the government does a good job, I'll be grateful; if the government doesn't do a good job, then I won't be grateful.' A shopkeeper, angry that the government is not helping them, responds, 'What's there to be grateful for?' An old man is more straightforward: 'Grateful my arse!'

On 9 March, Zhang Zhan begins to survey people's views on the residential lockdown. She asks every resident she encounters: 'Do you support the government's management methods?' The majority do not. One man responds, 'My wife and I are over seventy and we haven't received any help from the neighbourhood committee. We can't collect our pensions, we can't buy anything; you tell me if I support them.'

Zhang Zhan calls these opinions the 'true voice of China'. She finds them enormously encouraging and decides upon more direct confrontation.

By now, a fence has been erected around all four sides of the Old Railway Station neighbourhood, with only one small passageway in and out. When no one is entering or leaving, 'Red Armbands' block the passage with a one metre by one metre gate on wheels. In Zhang Zhan's eyes, the gate is a symbol of enslavement.

On 14 March, Zhang Zhan begins to attack the gate. She walks up to the Red Armbands and says in a loud voice, 'This is illegal. You have no right to restrict my freedom.' The Red Armbands surround her. Standing in their midst, Zhang Zhan delivers an impassioned speech on rights and freedom and denounces the hardships brought by the lockdown. As she is declaiming, she hears the Red Armbands muttering 'troublemaker', 'outrageous'.

The police rush to the scene. Just as they are about to reach her, Zhang Zhan shouts, 'I want to destroy this barrier.' There is a crashing noise as the gate hits the ground.

In the following days, Zhang Zhan pushes the gate down daily. The Red Armbands call the police and she lectures them on freedom and the evil of enslavement, not holding back her anger towards the government. 'Why must the news be fake?' 'Why must fascist methods be employed?'

Day by day, the police and the Red Armbands gradually lose patience. On 16 March, a Red Armband threatens to tie her up with rope and give her the boot. A few days later a policeman bellows, 'I will beat you to death!'

Zhang Zhan is not intimidated: 'Come on! Beat me! Call in more officers! Send me to prison!'

The policeman has no orders from higher authorities so he gruffly commands two police officers to escort her back to her hotel. Zhang Zhan resists. As the policewomen tug on her more forcefully, she becomes unsteady on her feet and sits down in the middle of the road. Everyone looks at her stonily. At that moment, Zhang Zhan suddenly feels at a loss. *Heavens*, she thinks, *what am I doing?*

'Look at yourself.' The policeman's voice is scornful. 'Are you any different from a shrew?'

It's a sharp rebuke. Zhang Zhan makes no reply. She raises her head, looks at the people surrounding her and stands up, bewildered, as if suddenly waking from a dream and unable to muster the energy to rebel.

It is a moment of realisation. Despite being in the midst of an act of resistance, she feels embarrassed at her ungraceful behaviour.

Yet she carries on fighting with the gate. Through Wuhan's cherry blossom season, Zhang Zhan doesn't notice the lonely flowers blooming.

The Red Armbands no longer inform the police, nor fend off her attacks. On 24 March she approaches the gate and shouts: 'If you don't represent justice and truth, you have no significance or value.' The guards do not respond. 'Today I want to represent justice and truth, because in today's China, the most important thing is not physical health, it is justice and truth.'

The gate comes down with a bang. A Red Armband listlessly raises his head to ask: 'Are you finished?' Zhang Zhan says she is finished. 'Well,' he sighs, 'if you're finished, then you can go back to your room.'

Zhang Zhan's speeches are not very convincing. No one in the Old Railway Station residential district knows what she means by justice and truth. When, like Don Quixote, she attacks the red-and-white gate again and again, the local residents look at her indifferently and say nothing. To be sure, some consider her irrational but in this city, with several million prisoners, Zhang Zhan is the only person pushing over gates, the only person battling the neighbourhood lockdown.

*

There are two propaganda posters on the wall of Imperial Ministry of Revenue Lane in the Wuchang district of Wuhan. One is white with a pair of giant handcuffs below which is written in red: 'Manufacturing rumours or spreading rumours will not escape the law.' The other poster is yellow: 'Create rumours, spread rumours. Punishable by law.'

In Wuhan there are millions of posters like that. Citizens hurry past, pretending not to see the threatening words, but they can't help thinking about Dr Li Wenliang. 'This sort of stuff is truly disgusting,' says a middle-aged man, pointing at a poster. 'That Li Wenliang, was what he said rumours? If we'd acted on what he had said, Wuhan would not be like this now.'

After the public fury surrounding Dr Li Wenliang's death on 7 February, the Chinese government promises to investigate in an attempt to rescue its image. On 19 March, a report is released. It casually mentions the incident, saying the law enforcement procedure was flawed, meaning that there was nothing wrong with the reprimand itself and that the police officers should have just been a bit smarter.

Zhang Zhan is furious. On 23 March, she slips out of the residential district and walks into the Zhongnan Road police station. Under the slogan painted on a wall – 'Strict justice, equitable enforcement' – she calmly asks the police: 'Why did you reprimand Li Wenliang?' They do not answer, nor does she expect them to. 'I did that to protest, to protest a country lacking justice,' she writes in an article.

Three days later, the pandemic seems to be under control. According to the government, there have been no new cases for three consecutive days. Zhang Zhan pushes over the gate and confronts the police and the Red Armbands one more time. She feels finally victorious, walking through the checkpoint in broad daylight. On

YouTube she calls her victory 'Crossing the road to freedom'.

She makes her way to the Wuhan No. 7 Hospital, where she observes the entrance for over two hours. She wants to know if the situation is as optimistic as the government is saying. 'There were still feverish patients arriving,' she says, 'and that was just one hospital. Could Wuhan really have zero new cases?'

When chatting with friends, Zhang Zhan says the number of people in China who died of coronavirus could not possibly be just the few thousand the government says, it has to be at least 100,000, though she admits she has no proof. 'You know their numbers are lies. If you investigated and compiled statistics, in the end all you'd be able to prove is the size of the lie, but what's the point of that?'

On 27 March, Zhang Zhan posts an essay on social media titled 'Cause of death is not that simple', in which she calls the Communist Party an evil cult and makes veiled references to biological weapons and massacres. She hints to her readers that it's possible the Communist Party deliberately released the novel coronavirus as a biological weapon.

This time, however, almost no one supports her viewpoint. At a gathering in early May, a friend criticises Zhang Zhan for peddling a conspiracy theory. Zhang Zhan responds with the 'beneficiary' argument: 'Who is the biggest beneficiary of this pandemic? It's the Communist Party, it uses the pandemic to strengthen its totalitarian rule.'

Zhang Zhan is right about that. Not long after the epidemic broke out, the Communist Party rolled out its 'rule by QR code'. First in Zhejiang and then nationwide, every Chinese citizen has to live a QR-code life. They must swipe their own QR code to get on a bus, a subway or a taxi, and at train stations and restaurants, informing the government of their whereabouts at all times. It's a new technology George Orwell hadn't thought of. Few people in China openly object. 'I really don't understand why nobody is talking about this,' says Zhang Zhan. 'It's such a serious issue, because with this thing, can the Chinese people have any privacy or any freedom?'

Perhaps because Zhang Zhan is posting words like this, the government begins to restrict her movements severely. Once again, she is unable to leave the residential district. Four people are always closely on her tail, following her, observing her. She persistently works to win over the four tails, hoping they will understand why she does what she does. It is all in vain. They continue to watch her, restrict her movements and occasionally manhandle her. It's disheartening. 'Shouldn't they have stood with me? Why were they doing that to me?' Zhang Zhan makes several attempts to break out and on one occasion succeeds, crashing through a checkpoint to get to a main street. Very soon, the four tails catch up with her, grab her four limbs, and carry her back in full view of startled bystanders.

'Completely senseless,' sighs Zhang Zhan. 'But I ought to forgive them.'

This goes on for about a week until 3 April, when, unable to endure any more, Zhang Zhan goes on a hunger strike in protest. The Red Armbands probably do not want to see her starve to death in front of them, so they finally loosen the restrictions on her. At noon on 4 April, after thirty-six hours of her hunger strike, Zhang Zhan drags her battered wheelie suitcase out of the Old Railway Station residential district, without the least bit of reluctance. It is not just the police and the Red Armbands that disappoint her, it is also the apathetic residents. 'I was fighting for their rights, but they had no reaction whatsoever.'

Zhang Zhan has read the Declaration of Independence and holds Thomas Jefferson in high esteem. In her view, people who live under tyrannical rule, like the worthy founders of the American republic, should charge through enemy lines in the battle for freedom. Yet in China she can't see any trace of defiance. 'They know the whole country is rotten to the core,' she writes in an article, 'yet they only think about their own lives. Why can't they manifest the slightest hint of resistance?'

'This world is too far from my ideal world,' says Zhang Zhan. After a moment's silence, she goes on: 'Perhaps that's because I have never lived in the real world.'

*

For many Chinese Christians, Zhang Zhan does not qualify as a 'limb of the Lord's body' – she rarely proselytises and rarely quotes the Bible in her essays. Sometimes she talks of the Good Samaritan, but her version is unlike the parable Jesus told. After her baptism in 2015, Zhang Zhan changed churches three times. All three churches disapproved of her struggles. 'I heard that they are afraid to even talk to me because of the things I have done,' says Zhang Zhan. 'My only companion is the Bible.'

In 2018 a priest told her, 'If you die because of the regime, it's a waste. Only if you die for the Lord will the Lord truly commemorate you.' Zhang Zhan had a big argument with the priest and stormed out. In her view, the true gospel goes beyond the words in the Bible. Helping people escape their suffering is far more important, and in China the suffering has a common origin, the Chinese Communist Party. 'I exist for the great cause of opposing communism,' she says. 'I have no other plans for this life, it's the only thing I want to do.'

This is the true reason Zhang Zhan went to Wuhan, clear-eyed about the likely consequences. Over the course of 104 hard days, she constantly thinks about her own death and the ways to die – poisoned, beaten to death, hit by a car, or perhaps one of the ways mentioned in the Bible, such as Jesus on the cross or Saint Steven stoned to death. She lives in constant fear, but is determined to carry on. 'If I actually die, the Lord will know why I died.'

On 8 April the Wuhan lockdown is rescinded, but Zhang Zhan has no intention of leaving. She believes the pandemic is just beginning and the disaster will become much worse. She wants to continue investigating, searching, visiting. She enters hospital wards, mixes with crowds of people, and ventures to police stations and public security bureaux to ask the police the whereabouts of Fang Bin. Her efforts are futile.

Zhang Zhan visits the Biandanshan cemetery on 26 April. She sees many new graves, including a tombstone with a one-line memorial for a senior citizen surnamed Tian who caught coronavirus and died because 'no medical treatment was available'. The person who commissioned the tombstone expressed the hope that future generations will not forget. Zhang Zhan posts a photograph online, praying, 'I hope officials do not destroy [this tombstone] and let it exist peacefully to be a record of this world.'

Through her friends, Zhang Zhan gets to know several families of people who succumbed to the novel coronavirus, including Jin Feng, who lost her husband, and Yang Min, who lost her daughter. She records Yang Min's battle and posts her words online. She visits Jin Feng's home and helps her fight for her rights. Jin Feng later sends Zhang Zhan a text message expressing her gratitude. Zhang Zhan is moved. 'That made me feel my work has some value. I didn't really do anything, but it inadvertently spread some light and unexpectedly brought warmth to another person. It lit me up too.'

By May, Wuhan is becoming warmer by the day. Zhang Zhan walks the streets sweating. She posts daily essays and videos on social media, reminding Chinese people not to forget the disaster. 'History repeats itself. Unfortunately, when people hear the deafening ring of the bell of history, they always pretend to hear nothing.'

On 14 May, Zhang Zhan goes to the Sanmin residential compound where another outbreak has occurred. She films workers locking down the district and adds her commentary: 'Fear of the virus and fear of the truth lead to lockdowns.'

Those are the final words she posts on social media. The next day Zhang Zhan's family receives a 'detention notification'. Time of arrest: 13.30 on 15 May 2020. Reason for arrest: picking quarrels and provoking trouble. Place of custody: Shanghai Pudong New District Detention Centre. No one knows how Zhang Zhan travelled the 800 kilometres from Wuhan to Shanghai.

Zhang Zhan always knew this day would come. 'I think they'll soon arrest me,' she'd said in April, 'and this time it will be tough, for sure.'

Shortly before her arrest, Zhang Zhan attended a gathering at a friend's home. It was a rare happy day. She ate fish, chicken and rice, and even had a little to drink. She told friends she is 'whole-heartedly seeking death'. 'I don't mind being a martyr,' she said. 'If the price of fighting tyranny is death, then I will gladly die.' She places two hands on a table, slightly embarrassed. 'But no matter what, I hope that while I'm alive, I will still love this world and still love these people.'

After Zhang Zhan is arrested, life in China becomes ever more difficult and the freedoms ordinary people enjoy are drastically reduced. In the following days, the pandemic surges in the west in Urumqi, Xinjiang, in the north-east in Tonghua, Jilin province, and in Shijiazhuang and Xingtai near Beijing. The Chinese government continues to employ its 'Wuhan experience' with a vengeance, locking down cities and halting transportation. People's homes are frequently sealed as layer upon layer of official paper slips are pasted one over another. Anyone who dares to defy the movement bans is heavily fined, abused, beaten and even tied to a tree as an example to the public. Countless people suffer shortages, but they seem incapable of uttering any sound.

Four months after her arrest, the prosecutor's office in Shanghai's Pudong New District forwards Zhang Zhan's indictment to the court. 'The accused used words and videos on internet social media such as Twitter and YouTube to distribute a large amount of fake information. She accepted interviews by foreign media. She maliciously hyped the novel coronavirus pneumonia epidemic. The audience was large, the negative influence was severe.'

It's hard to say when Zhang Zhan began her hunger strike, but she must have held out for a long time. On 17 December her lawyer finally sees her after overcoming numerous hurdles. She appears 'unrecognisably thin'. Her face is ashen and wrinkled and she wobbles when she walks.

For the duration of the visit, Zhang Zhan's hands are tied to her waist and a force-feeding tube is in her nose. Her lawyer implores her to resume eating, but Zhang Zhan is resolute. 'I will use hunger strikes to express the strongest non-cooperation with my evil persecution.'

On 28 December, the court convicts Zhang Zhan of 'the crime of picking quarrels and provoking trouble' and sentences her to four years in jail. She wears a pink down jacket and is restrained in a wheelchair. Although her hands are cuffed behind her and a cable is tied around her waist, she appears calm. She raises her head in the solemn courtroom to look at the golden national emblem and the imposing judges and prosecutors. 'This court is trying you, not me,' she says to the chief judge in her clear, gentle voice. 'When you put me into the accused dock, doesn't your conscience tell you this is wrong?'

In her 104 days in Wuhan, Zhang Zhan fought a battle knowing there was no prospect of victory, yet she still charged onto the battlefield. In the coming months and years, she will face more challenges, more tears and blood. But the words and images she leaves behind cannot be extinguished. In the midst of an earth-shattering calamity, a solitary woman pushed over the gate again and again.

6.

Just like boarding Noah's Ark

'Something must have happened,' thinks Li Xuewen.

It is the first day of 2020. Xuewen has just read a now-infamous news item on his mobile phone. The Wuhan Public Security Bureau has 'according to the law, investigated and dealt with' eight doctors for 'spreading rumours'. Xuewen puts down his mobile phone and ponders the backstory to this news item. 'The police would not do this of their own accord. They must have been following orders from higher-ups. And the higher-ups must have been following orders from even higher up. What are they trying to achieve?'

'I'm not a doctor. I didn't know how dangerous this virus is, but I take note of what the government does,' he explains. 'If the government metes out a light punishment, it won't be anything serious. But if they arrest people and show them on TV, that indicates it's something big.'

Xuewen was born in 1977. He is medium height and very slim, giving him a malnourished appearance. When he smiles, his mouth is a little lopsided, though he rarely smiles. He is always serious, and even when chatting he uses big words like totalitarianism, civil society, democracy and human rights. After completing a master's degree in 2008, he worked as a university teacher and an editor in a publishing company. He didn't keep these jobs for long, he believes because his articles critical of the government were published overseas.

His wife Huang Simin is a well-known lawyer who has represented many people in sensitive and at times dangerous political cases. Like Xuewen's articles, these cases bring no benefit to their lives, only torment. Local governments shun them, and they are forced to move frequently – from Wuhan to Guangzhou and Foshan in the south, then back to Wuhan. Along the way, the police summon them many times. The plight of a wanderer's life leads Xuewen to see the regime more clearly – no matter what the government says, you always need to be vigilant.

From that moment at the start of 2020, Xuewen began nagging people. 'Whenever I met anyone, I'd say it, I'd say it to my family and friends, I'd say to taxi drivers: "Take adequate protection, wear a mask." But no one paid me any attention.' He shakes his head. 'Chinese people believe government propaganda. Can't do anything about it.'

The government's disinformation that January – 'no human-to-human transmission', 'preventable and controllable', 'no need to panic' – causes countless people who could have avoided it, to be infected with a serious disease. It causes the whole world to be dragged down into an abyss. Although Xuewen senses danger, he does not fully realise the severity of the situation. He goes about his routine, attending social gatherings and, on 9 January, even accompanies Huang Simin to visit a friend at Tongji Hospital.

By then Tongji Hospital already has many infection cases, but Xuewen does not feel it is particularly risky. He observes that the hospital lobby is as crowded as a Sunday market and comments with a slight sense of superiority: 'I really have to admire the bravery of the people of Wuhan. There's an endless flow of people yet very few are wearing masks. This group psychology provides food for thought.'

By 20 January, the government reluctantly admits the novel coronavirus is 'human-to-human transmissible'. The words reverberate through the air of Wuhan like heavy artillery shells. 'Overnight, Wuhan went on a war footing,' says Xuewen. 'And that was the moment I decided to take my family and flee Wuhan.'

He spends quite a lot of time defending his escape. 'Isn't saving oneself a human right? Is it wrong for someone who lives in a totalitarian country and is deprived of truth to save himself? I am actually a victim ...' He keeps saying, 'I do not have a guilty conscience, I have no regrets.'

Those words do not seem convincing. Deep down, he probably wanted to stay in Wuhan to face the hardship with his fellow citizens, with his friends and neighbours. 'Had I stayed,' he mutters to himself, 'I could have done more.' He raises his head and speaks resolutely, 'But I have no regrets.'

He books flights out of Wuhan for three days later. Simin is in Thailand on business, so Xuewen intends to take her parents and her aged grandmother with him on the escape.

But the situation is far worse than he anticipated. Very early on the morning of 23 January, several friends inform Xuewen that Wuhan is going into lockdown. 'You probably won't be able to leave.'

It's 2 am. Xuewen springs out of bed and calls his wife in Thailand to tell her to change the flights for the whole family. He then tries many car hire apps to get him over to his in-laws' house, but none respond. After half an hour, he finally manages to get a car to drive him the five kilometres.

The city resembles a ghost town. Along the way, he passes several silent neighbourhoods usually bustling with dressed-up young people and noisy music into the wee hours. But in the early hours of 23 January, Xuewen sees not a single person and hears nothing but the sound of the gentle breeze. 'Even the streetlights were cold,' he later writes. His is the only car on the road, as if he is traversing an enormous, deserted cemetery. He can't help feeling afraid. 'It was beyond belief. It was a completely surreal scene. I'd never seen Wuhan like that,' he says, his fear still lingering.

He asks the driver to wait downstairs while he dashes into his in-laws' home. Without allowing for any discussion, he tells them Wuhan is about to go into lockdown. 'Grab all your cash, carry what you can and let's go, straight away.'

Simin's grandmother, Xiong Qiaoyun, is eighty-five. She lived through the Japanese invasion and the infamous bombing of Wuhan and can never forget the times in her childhood when she had to evacuate. Seventy-five years later, her city again descends into crisis. Tottering out of her home and looking up the empty street, she can't help thinking, *Golly, this is just like the escape from the Japanese invaders.*

Possibly out of his own fear, the driver hasn't waited for them. Xuewen returns to the car hire app but this time it is even harder. The app's maps show not a single car available within ten kilometres of their location in the centre of Wuhan. The little group look at each other in dismay; no, in terror of the approaching apocalypse. A taxi in the distance approaches. Xuewen frantically waves his arms and shouts, but the driver doesn't seem to hear and speeds past. 'What's going on?' his mother-in-law asks in horror. 'Why is this happening?'

It isn't until 4 am that they find a taxi. Arriving at the airport feels like jumping from a prehistoric era to modern-day Times Square in New York. 'The whole city was desolate and in darkness, then all of sudden we were in a noisy, bustling, brightly lit place. It was mind-boggling.'

Just as they arrive at the airport, the freeway behind them is sealed off. The lockdown has begun.

The airport is chaotic. They can't find a single member of staff and have no way of knowing when their plane will take off. More and more people crowd into the terminal, rushing about and shouting in desperation at unattended check-in counters. Everyone looks terrified. At about 6 am, the airport staff begin to stream in. They wear thick face masks. Like a phalanx of ice-cold robots, they are expressionless and unresponsive to questioning.

'International flights ceased but domestic flights operated as usual. I have no idea why,' says Xuewen. 'There were no checks when we boarded, no temperature checks. Our eighty-five-year-old maternal grandmother was not even asked to sign a disclaimer, which is usually required. I don't know whether they forgot.'

As the plane taxis down the runway, Xuewen finally calms down. 'It was like we boarded Noah's Ark,' he says. By then it is getting light; in the warm glow of dawn, the lakes of Wuhan are as smooth as a mirror and flowers quietly bloom. In the crowded hospital wards people are dying in agony, while others wait in panic to face their own hard times. 'I was not happy; on the contrary, I had a heavy heart. I might have escaped but behind me was a black hole,' says Xuewen gravely. 'A black hole with eleven million people.'

*

'You're just selfish trash.'
'You'll end up in hell.'
'I hope the virus gets you.'

On social media, escapees from Wuhan are being reviled. When he sees these posts, Xuewen and his family are hiding in an apartment in Guangzhou. They never greet their neighbours, fearing they will reveal they've come from Wuhan. 'At that time everyone treated people from Wuhan and Hubei like dogs that had to be beaten,' says Xuewen indignantly.

The next day is Lunar New Year's Eve. Xuewen prepares some dishes with his in-laws – vegetables, mushrooms and a tureen of lotus root soup. They eat the food, drink some alcohol and repeat some of the usual auspicious sayings. But Xuewen is gloomy. He posts a number of tweets on Twitter, describing his escape from Wuhan and criticising the hasty and sloppy lockdown. ‘Such a sudden lockdown was irresponsible. How were millions of people supposed to live? Our family and friends are there.’

His tweets incite a tidal wave of abuse. Several months later it still rankles. ‘They viciously cursed me, but what had I done wrong?’ He calls the people who curse him ‘little pinkies’: young people who idolise the Communist Party and are led astray by its propaganda. On closer examination, it’s not just little pinkies; many others accuse Xuewen of ‘spreading the virus’.

The Chinese government later congratulates itself for its ‘victory over the virus’, suggesting the whole world should emulate the ‘Chinese way’. The heavy price paid by the Chinese people, especially the people of Wuhan, is passed over. According to some Chinese scholars, the Confucian cultural influence conditions East Asian people to obey authority and adopt a collective perspective rather than a Western individualistic one. So East Asian people obey instructions to wear masks because they worry less about themselves and more about their families and neighbourhoods. If the theory is true, the ‘great victory over the virus’ does not belong to the Chinese government but to the modesty and self-discipline of the Chinese people.

For Xuewen, this theory helps clear up the confusion in his mind. If the Chinese people revere collectivism, his escape from Wuhan does not deserve praise because it was a self-interested act rather than a collectivist one. He did not consider the safety of others.

Several days after arriving in Guangzhou, Xuewen catches a severe cold and coughs incessantly. 'At the time, I really thought I was infected and wondered whether I ought to isolate, and I worried about how I would get to a hospital in Guangzhou.' His mind would naturally have darker thoughts, about death – and the torrent of criticism and abuse. As he reads posts on Weibo and WeChat about the surge of cases in Wuhan, about the wailing, struggling and the number of deaths, none of his own dark thoughts seem to matter anymore. 'It really was like a scene from hell. It was so painful.'

Xuewen is fast asleep when his friend's frantic phone call comes. Hu Weili is a teacher. Her father has cancer and has contracted the novel coronavirus in the hospital where he is undergoing treatment. That was on 18 January, when the government was saying the novel coronavirus was not transmissible from human to human. After her father returned home, with no instructions to take preventative measures, his wife, daughter and daughter-in-law are infected, one after another. On 27 January, the day Premier Li Keqiang pays a visit to Wuhan, four members of the family are now infected. On the TV, Li Keqiang promises that all patients who should be admitted to hospital will be admitted. However, the reality is that no matter how hard she tries, Hu Weili is unable to have her father admitted to a hospital.

'Hu Weili rarely contacts me. If she weren't desperate, she wouldn't have sought me out,' says Xuewen. 'At that time the hospital system in Wuhan had collapsed so it was virtually impossible to find a hospital bed. I didn't know if I would be able to help so I got her to write a plea for help which I circulated to my friends on social media.'

Every word, every punctuation mark, of Hu Weili's three-hundred-character plea bares her desperation.

> *Please save my family! I've been feverish for three days. My mother and my sister-in-law also have a fever. No one is helping – we've been told to wait at home and are not permitted to leave the house. That means we will die at home. We make phone calls, but they do nothing, they do nothing for confirmed novel coronavirus patients! We have three young children here! How can we live like this? How? Please help us!*

Weili's plea quickly spreads on Weibo where it is read and reposted by even more people, including several newspapers in Beijing. Within a few hours, Hu Weili telephones Xuewen again to request he delete her post.

'At first, she requested me to circulate her plea, then she wanted me to delete it. I asked her what was going on. It turned out the police had visited her at her home in the Qingshan district. The police said, "If you delete it, your father can go to hospital tomorrow. If you don't delete it, then you'll just have to wait."'

Xuewen does not analyse why the police act this way, but anyone who has lived in China would not be surprised. According to the logic of the Chinese government, Hu Weili's cry for help is 'negative news', suggesting the government is incompetent, ineffective and indifferent to human life. The government takes extreme measures to suppress 'negative news'. Officials issue a stream of prohibiting orders to the media and many people are summoned, reprimanded and warned. An army of vigilant keyboard warriors is unleashed to make a huge ruckus. In the midst of the pandemic, the Chinese government is more concerned about 'negative news' than the virus.

Xuewen tells Hu Weili and the police officers standing next to her as she makes the call, 'I can delete the post, but the information has already been circulated widely and no one can completely delete it.' The police stay in Hu Weili's home, threatening her and watching over her as she makes endless phone calls requesting people to delete the post from their social media.

One of Xuewen's friends, the poet Ye Kuangzheng who lives in Beijing, is a Weibo 'Big V' – a verified internet influencer. He had reposted and commented on Hu Weili's plea, resulting in more reposts and more commentary. He too is harassed by the police. 'At 2 am the police called Ye Kuangzheng demanding he delete the post,' says Xuewen, shaking his head. 'They're just that shameless, and there's nothing you can do.'

The Hu Weili incident ends well. The police fulfil their promise. The next day they arrange for her father to check into a hospital. By posting then deleting Hu Weili's plea, Xuewen finally feels he has done something good for Wuhan. 'Hu Weili later said I had saved her father's life,' Xuewen says with a rare smile, though he soon reverts to a serious demeanour. 'I didn't actually do anything.'

More than the virus, Xuewen hates the regime that conceals the truth and suppresses all voices but its own. On 28 January he writes on his WeChat page, 'I don't know how many more of the people back home will die in silence, they are not even counted.' Late one night soon after, he posts a photo of a group of Wuhan residents, their faces obscured. In the background is the Yellow Crane Tower, an ancient structure that has been standing on the bank of the Yangtze River since the third century. 'On that night,' Xuewen says, 'I heard the bitter wails of the people and the sound of the totalitarian edifice crumbling.' A day or two later, he posts: 'I can't write now. Even my outrage is coming up blank ... Festering, just festering ...'

*

When he opens the door, Xuewen is confronted with a dazzling white visage. Half a dozen people wearing white full-body PPE are there, with masks and protective goggles, looking like visitors from outer space. The one in charge examines Xuewen's ID card and takes the temperature of each family member. He then sends in a member of the team to spray disinfectant in every room.

Xuewen is nervous as he looks at the visitors from outer space; he knows exactly what will happen next. 'They were from the disease prevention department to spray disinfectant as an advance party for the police,' he explains. 'My family had come from Wuhan and even the police were scared.'

The police soon arrive. One is in uniform, probably from the local police station, to lead the way. Two others, one fat, one skinny, are plain-clothed. Xuewen calls them 'guobao', short for the Domestic Security Protection Command of the Public Security Bureau. Secret police. They monitor, interrogate, harass and even beat up those who dare challenge the communist regime. Although they rarely appear in public, they are no strangers to Xuewen and Simin. In the past decade, he has had many interactions with the guobao; none of them was pleasant.

The guobao ask Xuewen and Simin to 'go for a walk' with them. Their destination is not police headquarters or the local police station. It's the office of the building's management company downstairs. 'They were scared too and definitely didn't want us to go to the police station,' says Xuewen. 'Because I came from Wuhan.'

Simin is unwilling to cooperate. 'If you want to talk, then let's talk at a police station.' When they reach the downstairs office, a heated argument ensues. Simin insists on following 'legal process', which the two guobao firmly resist.

'I've never seen a lawyer like you,' the fat guobao bellows.

'I've never seen police like you,' Simin retorts.

It is 11 February and a cold winter's day in Guangzhou. Watching his wife argue vigorously with the guobao, Xuewen is somewhat amused. 'They were wearing masks, so their breath fogged up their glasses,' he recalls with a smile. 'However, I thought that arguing like that would solve nothing, so I put my hand on her arm to stop her and said to those two guobao, "If you want to talk, go ahead and talk."'

Chinese law stipulates that this talk can be considered to be under summons, though it is slightly irregular. Xuewen and Simin sit on one side of the rudimentary office and the two guobao sit on the other side. The fat officer keeps a record. The skinny officer seems to be in charge. 'Do you know why we sought you out?' he asks.

Of course Xuewen knows why. Three days earlier he had set in motion a huge movement. He contacted all his friends in Wuhan. They set up social media accounts called 'Never Forget Li Wenliang' to campaign to have a bronze statue of the doctor cast and put on display.

Discussing this several months later, Xuewen becomes very serious. 'I cried when Li Wenliang died. It was such an emotional event for me. I thought I and my circle of friends should stand up and do something for him.' He then quotes Dr Li Wenliang's famous words: 'A healthy society cannot have just one voice.'

The petition Xuewen posts is written in his serious and meticulous style.

> *Compatriots, we are Wuhan citizens in various professions who care about social justice. Like everyone, we were shocked when Doctor Li Wenliang died late in the evening of the 6th of February 2020. We felt tremendous grief and anger. Our consciences compel us to do something ... To memorialise him, to commemorate his bravery in speaking out, and to put the spirit of his words into practice, we have started a fundraising campaign for a bronze statue of Li Wenliang.*

They envisage a huge statue on a plinth big enough to engrave with the words of the police reprimand.

'Li Wenliang represents honour, and he also represents humiliation,' says Xuewen, raising his head, a sharp look in his eyes, his facial muscles twitching. 'We want the world to remember his honour and his humiliation for eternity.'

He posts his petition on WeChat as well as Twitter and Facebook. The public response is immediate. Within hours more than 30,000 RMB (A$6300) is deposited in the donation account. Someone even tells Xuewen that he is willing to fully fund the statue himself. Xuewen declines the offer. 'It was not a question of funding. It was in essence a citizens' movement. We wanted as many people to participate as possible.'

The government pays close attention to the movement. A day later, the petition is being deleted from social media within China's 'Great Firewall' and the police warn Xuewen's friends in Wuhan. Even the people who repost the petition are harassed by the police. Xuewen knows there is no chance he will escape. 'I instigated the movement, so there could be no escape. But I was prepared.'

Xuewen's claim to be prepared is probably intended to boost his morale, because there is no way to prepare; he has no idea what will happen next. 'Being "invited to drink tea" is a certainty, arrest is possible; as for imprisonment ...' He shakes his head. 'I thought about it, but I felt there was only a small chance of that.'

The chat on 11 February lasts an hour. In the face of guobao interrogation, Xuewen maintains his composure. He doesn't know who initiated the movement or who wrote the proposal. He is unwilling to sign a record of interview. In fact, his response to almost every question is 'I don't know', 'I'm unclear about that', or 'I don't remember'.

The skinny guobao holds a stack of paper in front of Xuewen's face that includes a printout of his post on Twitter. 'Is this person you?'

'Of course it isn't me. That person is called Siwen. My name is Li Xuewen. How could it be the same person?'

'So, you dare to do it, but don't dare to admit it's you?' asks the skinny guobao sarcastically.

'If so, yes; if not, no,' Xuewen responds calmly. 'How is daring involved?'

'Actually, Siwen is my account name,' Xuewen says later, adding with satisfaction, 'If I'm going to admit it, I definitely would not admit it to them, right?' He pauses and his demeanour becomes serious. 'This is my freedom of speech as a citizen. They have no right to interfere.

'My chief concern was that they would use the pandemic as an excuse to lock us up or force us out of our home. They threatened to force us out if we even mentioned Li Wenliang's name or accepted media interviews. At that time, people from Hubei province were virtually unable to go anywhere.'

Xuewen is now worried sick. 'I had a family to feed so there was no choice. I had to agree to their demands.'

For many days after the interview, Xuewen is under virtual house arrest. He is allowed to walk around the apartment complex but is absolutely prohibited from leaving the neighbourhood. One day he wants to go out to buy a pack of cigarettes. The police officers on duty prevent him from exiting the building. 'Get someone else to buy it for you,' they say.

Right up until April, Xuewen rarely posts anything on social media. The guobao harass him almost weekly. They occasionally make a big scene, at other times less so. 'They came to interview me six times and took written records on three occasions,' says Xuewen. 'Under those circumstances, I couldn't do anything, I couldn't say anything. I could only watch as the situation deteriorated by the day. It was really depressing.'

According to the guobao, Xuewen's proposal for a statue was intended to 'stir up' the Li Wenliang incident. In the communist regime's terminology, this means 'exaggerating and embellishing Li Wenliang's influence, inciting discontent of the people, with the purpose of opposing the communist regime'. However, some twenty days after Xuewen's petition, to the surprise of many, the Chinese government begins to propagandise the Li Wenliang incident. Newspapers publish reports on and in praise of Dr Li, who now becomes an 'outstanding person'.

In September he is posthumously awarded an official May Fourth Medal. Hubei province honours him at a large-scale commemorative event, and the provincial Party Secretary Ying Yong includes Li Wenliang when he praises 'heroic martyrs', describing them as the 'most beautiful people of the new era' and 'the backbone of the nation'.

As the Communist Party goes all out to praise Dr Li, the writer who initiated the memorial to Li Wenliang is hiding in an apartment in Guangzhou – dispirited, harassed by the police, effectively a prisoner.

That the Communist Party's words and its actions don't match up is not really news. When Dr Li Wenliang dies, they fear him; then later they use him. Everything they do is designed to turn Li Wenliang into a communist hero, rather than a people's hero. If he is going to be a martyr, he can only be a communist martyr and not a martyr persecuted by the Communist Party. In the end, this young doctor – reprimanded and berated for posting medical information to his friends – died in the line of duty. To add to his misfortune, he becomes a part of the Communist Party's 'victory' over the pandemic.

After Li Wenliang dies, his Weibo account becomes sacred. Countless people leave messages, commemorating him and telling him everything on their minds. They bare their souls, revealing to him things they would never tell anyone else. By December 2020, Dr Li's first Weibo post has more than one million comments. 'Dr Li, it's winter. Is it cold where you are?' 'Dr Li, you won't be reprimanded in heaven, will you?' 'Dr Li, I split up with my boyfriend today. I'm very sad.'

Some commentators say Li Wenliang's Weibo account has become the Chinese people's 'Wailing Wall'. Xuewen says perhaps this is a realisation of what he had attempted – millions of people using their tears and inner voices to erect a virtual stele as a record of Dr Li's honour as well as his humiliation.

On 25 April, the life of exile for Xuewen and his family ends and they return to Wuhan. The plane lands late at night. Xuewen knits his brow as he looks over this city that has been plagued with misfortunes.

'I've been depressed recently. Perhaps I should force myself to write something,' he says to friends at a social gathering. However, he seems unable to pull himself together. He doesn't publish anything. He is always frowning, frowning as he observes Wuhan and China.

At times he is more optimistic: 'I can hear the sound of the totalitarian edifice crumbling.' At other times he is dejected because the catastrophe is not over, and it could become worse. He is concerned about the dissidents who are being persecuted – Zhang Jialong, Ou Biaofeng, Du Bin and the unyielding Zhang Zhan. After Zhang Zhan is imprisoned, Xuewen boasts to his friends: 'The first thing I did upon returning to Wuhan was to take Zhang Zhan out for a meal. She was happy that day and told me it was the best meal she'd had in Wuhan for several months.'

On 28 December 2020, the day Zhang Zhan is sentenced, Xuewen is sad and indignant. He writes a long poem.

You pushed your way through this city of fear
Your exhaustion and tenacity
Tore back the veil concealing so many lies
...
Your body is shackled with manacles and leg-irons
But your soul is forever free
No one can put you on trial
Those who try you
Will themselves be put on trial.

The sentiment is defiant, but Xuewen is dispirited. His determination flags with each passing day. 'My path to redemption has been so difficult,' he tells a group of friends late one night. 'Sometimes I'm at the edge of mental collapse.'

By then, he and Simin are divorced. He lives alone in a small apartment and rarely goes out. He often just stares blankly at the walls.

He says his divorce and the pandemic are not connected. 'There were cracks in our relationship much earlier,' he says, as if discussing a piece of porcelain. At other times he admits the scars caused by the pandemic have not healed. 'They make grief even more painful, and a shattered relationship more shattered.'

'After returning to Wuhan, I have come to feel the pandemic was not as bad as I initially feared. Look outside. The streets are very lively, but I can still distinctly feel this is no longer the Wuhan of before.'

Xuewen is sitting in a Wuhan restaurant on a stiflingly hot afternoon in May 2020 having afternoon tea with friends. Dust floating above him in the room resembles a shroud. 'I mean, the life we lived in the past has been ousted. It's as if a sharp knife cut our lives in half. One half is pre-coronavirus, the other half post-coronavirus. It's unlikely we will ever be able to go back to our past lives.'

He sets down his cutlery and wipes his mouth with a napkin. 'As for me, it's like' – he points to his chest – 'it's like there's a hole here.'

7.

The darkest moment

'There's a difference between catching this disease and not catching it, just as experiencing it in Wuhan or elsewhere is also different,' says Wang Gangcheng slowly. 'Some things have to be personally experienced to truly comprehend them.' He raises his right arm and rubs his nose with the back of his hand – not his fingers – and continues. 'For most of the people in Wuhan, it's nowhere near over. It's like being injured. Some wounds heal quickly, some take time, and some will never heal.'

Gangcheng is easily recognisable on the streets of Wuhan. He's 1.78 metres (5 feet 10 inches) tall, rather stout, and has an imposing gait, like a slowly advancing armoured vehicle. In his thirty-odd years, he has experienced few setbacks. He has followed a predictable path in life: gaining an education, joining the workforce, marrying as expected and having a child at the appropriate time. He hardly ever oversteps the bounds of what is proper. As a mid-level employee at a large company, he is not wealthy, but his income is higher than that of most Wuhan residents. His family life is warm and harmonious, despite occasional arguments. As for the future, he has little ambition and few worries. 'If it weren't for this year,' he says with a wistful smile, 'there wouldn't be anything remarkable about my life.

'Right up to the day of the lockdown I was calm and composed,' says Gangcheng. He heard about the eight doctors who had been 'dealt with according to the law' for 'fabricating and spreading rumours'. He didn't feel any of this was particularly important, although he knew the story of his friend Shao Shengqiang.

Shao is a moderately famous Wuhan entrepreneur. At thirty-one years old, he holds a position in the Communist Youth League, owns several enterprises – restaurants, a headhunting company, a bakery – and frequently contributes money and goods to charitable causes. He's a member of Wuhan's wealthy class who often boasts of his success. 'I own so many businesses.' 'For me, money is not an issue.'

On 3 January, as CCTV reported on the doctors 'spreading rumours', Shao's symptoms emerged: coughing, diarrhoea and a temperature of 39.7°C. Several days later he was diagnosed with 'pneumonia of unknown cause'. His condition soon deteriorated; his lungs began to fail;

the hospital issued a 'critical illness notification'. There was no officially endorsed treatment plan so intravenous immunoglobulin therapy was employed to save his life. It's an extremely expensive therapy – 250,000 RMB (A$50,500) over the course of a month.

But Gangcheng doesn't see how any of this could be connected to him. The government's messages – 'no human-to-human transmission', 'it's preventable and controllable' – gives him confidence. Those words make him feel completely assured. When he raises the issue of the new disease at home one day, his father chides him: 'There's a lot of keyboard warriors out there who are controlled by enemy forces. They're out to smear China, so don't let them lead you by the nose.' Gangcheng doesn't entirely endorse his father's opinion, but he doesn't reject it either.

Like many in the middle class, Gangcheng trusts the Chinese government and relies on it. China is a 'semi-democratic country' that is still developing, he says. If the government makes mistakes, it should be 'viewed in the light of development' – that is, with forgiveness and sympathy. He is amused by the vulgarity of the stupid politicians in the British satirical comedy *In the Loop*, commenting, 'That's probably close to the reality ... The West is not so good, and China is not so bad. Western society appears to be civilised but their murky deeds are not less than in China, and their despicable acts are even more despicable than China's.'

In mid-January, vigilant Wuhan residents begin to stock up on masks and alcohol sanitisers. Gangcheng thinks they're 'overreacting'.

On 18 January, he and his family go to the largest Walmart in Wuhan to buy necessities for the Lunar New Year season. The supermarket is crowded but few people wear masks and neither does Gangcheng. He thinks there's no need.

After he leaves the supermarket, a friend from outside the city asks, 'How's the situation in Wuhan?' Gangcheng responds casually, echoing Deng Xiaoping's promise about Hong Kong after the handover, 'Horses still run, dancers still dance.'

That day, while Gangcheng and his family are shopping in high spirits at Walmart, Shao Shengqiang is on oxygen in the Wuhan Union Hospital. He still struggles to breathe, although he has passed the most critical stage. He boosts his own morale by repeating to himself, 'I must be like a fighter.' He has observed the chaos and scenes of terror in the hospital. 'The intensive care wards were full ... On my floor, people died every day.'

The Chinese media do not report these grim facts. The leaders are as wise as ever, and the people are preparing to celebrate the Spring Festival. In the famous Baibuting neighbourhood, an enormous public banquet is underway. According to reports, over 40,000 families indulge in this mass banquet, gathering in banquet halls in a miasma of smoke and steam, applauding official speeches and sharing food from their plates. No precautions are taken despite the virus raging through the city. After the banquet, newspapers and television stations speak in unison in praise of the perfect and harmonious occasion.

Among Gangcheng's circle of friends on WeChat, the banquet occasions heated debate. 'People all over the country are worried about Wuhan but the people of Wuhan are unconcerned,' some say.

Gangcheng sees many posts like that. He describes the debate as 'a small-scale carnival' – these views are 'very unscientific' and 'very irrational'. Still, he's caught a cold; he coughs continuously. His friends bluntly ask, 'You're always coughing. Have you got the novel coronavirus?' Some urge him to go for a check-up at a hospital. Gangcheng stalls. He starts to check his own temperature regularly. He has two thermometers, one for his forehead and the other for inside his ear. He thinks both are inaccurate. 'The readings were going up and down, so I was always worried.' His wife Ah Hui teases him for behaving like a lunatic.

On 23 January he sleeps in so is late to hear the earthshattering news that the city is in lockdown. People rush to buy masks, alcohol sanitisers, food, vegetables, toilet paper – the shelves of supermarkets are stripped bare. Gangcheng claims he's not at all panicked – 'I was very calm.' He has booked a good restaurant for the family's New Year's Eve dinner, but he recognises that 'things may be getting serious, so we won't go out for that dinner'. He cancels the reservation and remains calm.

Gangcheng is unhurried as he talks of that time, playing down the seriousness of the situation, although his account of his feelings shifts. 'Thinking it over, I was in fact a little stunned. The situation abruptly changed and I just didn't have time to react. I really was a little stunned.'

Gangcheng eats his meals as usual, sleeps, chats with his family, but he remains in his 'a little bit stunned' state, like a child on a rumbling railway track watching a train speed towards him but not knowing what he ought to do.

*

Gangcheng's family celebrates New Year's Eve at home. They cook some dishes, open some wine, boil up some dumplings, then sit around the table to watch the CCTV gala. Gangcheng looks normal and even laughs a few times, but later he can't remember what he ate or watched. He's worried about many things. His parents are elderly and frail. His daughter is not yet two years old. He is the backbone of the family so he cannot collapse, and he cannot let his family see his apprehension.

He is also vaguely aware of changes in his body but prefers not to face up to them, and he is even less willing to think about the infectiousness of this disease.

'Starting on New Year's Eve I began to feel sick,' says Gangcheng. His cough becomes severe and his muscles ache. After he gets out of bed the next morning, he feels fatigued all over. 'I felt drained and had no appetite. I just wanted to sleep.' He repeatedly measures his temperature. It's normal, yet he is not reassured. At about ten in the evening, he measures his temperature again and finally sees a result he does not want to see – he has a fever. 'I didn't know whether I should go to hospital,' he says. 'I feared I really had it.' Gangcheng telephones his father, who insists he go to a hospital. But Gangcheng still hesitates.

The community disease prevention and control system has been implemented, under which the neighbourhood committee keeps track of patients and arranges for doctors' appointments. Gangcheng belongs to the Dongfang neighbourhood, whose highest official is a party member called Li Qiongli. She is the most famous person in the neighbourhood. Her hardworking, selfless and fearless style has been covered in many newspaper articles and TV reports, which valorise her as a superwoman, a hero of the common people.

But late in the evening of 25 January, Gangcheng is unable to get through to Party Secretary Li on the telephone. Feeling helpless, he phones the community doctor's number but the person on the other end is very cold: 'If you've got a fever then go to a hospital.'

He feels even more hopeless. ‘My mood at that time …’ Gangcheng shakes his head. ‘Apart from being ill, I was more concerned that if I really was infected with the novel coronavirus, it would definitely be a huge financial burden on my family.’

Gangcheng wavers again, then decides to go to the hospital.

The night is gloomy and cold. It’s raining. He coughs under an umbrella as he makes his way to the gate of his compound. He doesn’t encounter a single person; there’s not a soul on the street. Lights are on in every window, but he doesn’t hear a sound other than the fine rain on the ground. He’s worn out and despondent. Many feelings well up in his heart. ‘That scene,’ he says softly, ‘is something I’ll never forget.’

He drives to the nearby Red Cross Hospital, one of the first hospitals designated to treat the novel coronavirus in Wuhan. This is already an infraction of the rules because the government has prohibited private cars from going out on the road, but he can no longer worry about such things. By the time he arrives at the hospital it is almost 11 pm. He sees blue disaster relief tents, doctors wearing white PPE, patients and their deeply worried families rushing about, and flashing lights on police cars and ambulances parked by the side of the road. A man shouts irritably into a phone, ‘Hurry up! Hurry up!’

Gangcheng parks his car and follows the noise into the hospital lobby. Countless patients, many sitting on gaudily coloured plastic stools, are eating and sleeping in a snaking line. Some unoccupied stools have buns, bottles of water and the like perched on them. No one knows where the owners have gone; perhaps some will never return. In the coming days, in this hospital and others, Gangcheng encounters people who flop down on the ground and are unable to get up again. Onlookers gasp laments of regret but nobody seems surprised; death is no longer shocking.

*

Around this time Shao Shengqiang's condition has stabilised. On Lunar New Year's Eve he eats a simple hospital lunch and takes a shuttle bus from Wuhan Union Hospital to the Red Cross Hospital. As the bus passes through empty streets, Shao looks at his fellow patients and the evening sky, devoid of the usual fireworks. He is overcome with a wave of sadness and almost bursts into tears.

In the Red Cross Hospital his condition improves; he is elated. The next morning he circulates a government announcement to his friends on social media – in a manner befitting his role as a leader in the Communist Youth League – and comments, 'Centralised command

and planning is the most efficient. We don't want to panic and have chaos!' By that evening, about when Gangcheng's fever begins, Shao mentions a 'sister matron' who praised him as 'the most obedient and cooperative patient'. Deeply moved, Shao writes, 'It must be so hard for you nurses.'

*

Gangcheng nervously makes his way through the lobby, trying his best to steer clear of patients waiting for treatment. He finds the outpatient service specialising in fevers. A nurse aims a digital thermometer gun at his forehead: 36.8°C. 'You don't have a fever,' she tells Gangcheng. 'Go home.'

Gangcheng persists. 'That's impossible. I just measured myself and I was definitely feverish.' The nurse hesitates then produces a mercury thermometer. Gangcheng puts it under his arm.

A few minutes later the results are in. The nurse studies the reading and reflexively takes a step back. 'It's 38.3,' she tells Gangcheng, 'you really do have a fever.'

Several months later, Gangcheng still feels a lingering fear. 'If I hadn't persisted, if I had believed the nurse, I certainly would have gone home,' he mumbles. 'And once home there were my parents, my child ...' He laughs quietly. 'If that had happened, it possibly would be a very different story.'

A doctor instructs Gangcheng to go upstairs for a CT scan then bring the results back. When Gangcheng returns, the doctor says, 'You definitely have it. Look,' he gesticulates, 'here's some inflammation, and here too.' Gangcheng listens, only half-understanding. 'Your condition is not serious,' the doctor continues. 'No need to be hospitalised. I'll give you some medicine and you can go home to take it.'

It's now midnight. In an apartment not far away, Gangcheng's parents and Ah Hui are worried sick as they wait for news. Gangcheng walks out of the hospital with a heavy heart, but he also has a strange sense of relief. The thing that he has been worrying about has happened, as if a boulder suspended over his head for a long time has finally fallen. He no longer feels 'stunned'. He is very clear about what he must do – take his whole family to hospital to measure their temperatures and have CT scans, and avoid speaking to them as much as is possible. Then he must arrange for his wife and parents to move in together while he goes to his parents' home. 'I'm lucky because we have two apartments,' he says quietly.

Gangcheng once participated in an unusual corporate training event with a group of colleagues. He walked into a totally dark room. He could see nothing and lost his sense of direction. As he groped his way forward, a voice asked, 'Wang Gangcheng, what do you feel?' In the first week of self-isolation at his parents' home, Gangcheng feels as if he is back in that room.

He has no appetite, he coughs more and more violently, and he has high temperatures – as high as 38.8°C – at seemingly fixed times. He frequently retches but is unable to bring anything up; he leans over the washbasin in the kitchen, his body twitching as he howls like a wild animal. 'I'll never forget that feeling. It felt like I was going to vomit my own stomach up. Each time I felt I'd pass out if it happened again.' He suspects it is a side effect of the medicine as well as a symptom of the disease, but he can't be certain. He doesn't know if he should go back to the hospital.

One day he wakes up in the middle of the night because he feels the quilt cover is pressing uncomfortably on his chest. The covers are nowhere to be seen. 'That's a serious symptom, chest tightness and shortness of breath,' he says, still haunted. 'It's actually a bit dangerous.'

And there is his family. Although their temperatures and CT scan results are normal, Gangcheng does not feel reassured. Sometimes, he is certain he has infected them.

'Physical reactions are secondary, psychological fear is the most significant,' he says. 'In those circumstances, I knew nothing. I didn't know what kind of illness it was nor how to treat it. Even the doctors didn't know. I didn't know if I was going to ...' He doesn't continue.

He appears anxious, as if he's back in the pitch-dark training room. When that voice in the dark room asked, 'Wang Gangcheng, what do you feel?' his answer was, 'I can feel death.'

Gangcheng is not a melancholy person, but in the following three months tears flow from time to time. He cries for his family, he cries for his own difficult life, and he cries for total strangers. His psychology makes it difficult for him to utter the word 'cry'. Instead, he says 'emotional breakdown', as if this might make him appear less weak.

His first emotional breakdown occurs on 26 January, the first day of his self-isolation. Approaching noon, his father brings him lunch. To avoid passing on the infection, Gangcheng puts on a mask and opens all the windows. He stands in a corner as though he's on the edge of a minefield, keeping as far from his father as he can, as he watches him enter and take out a lunch box. After his father leaves, Gangcheng opens the lunch box and looks at the steaming hot food and two nicely browned spring onion flat cakes. Tears stream down his face.

'My father made it specially for me. He's so old and now he has to go to so much trouble, running around, and can still give thought to what I like to eat.'

While Gangcheng is silently sobbing, Wuhan is drowning in tears. Every hospital, every neighbourhood medical centre, is packed with patients in despair. A young girl chases after a truck transporting corpses, wailing, 'Mother, mother!' A forty-year-old daughter in tears asks a doctor on a telephone, 'My father has lost consciousness. What should I do?'

*

In the midst of the city's misery, Shao Shengqiang is back in high spirits. He posts a photograph of Dr Zhong Nanshan, with Dr Zhong's famous words: 'Wuhan will definitely get through this!' Zhong Nanshan is a household name in China. In 2003 he was called 'a leader in the battle against SARS'. Seventeen years later, he is the one who tells the media – on the orders of higher authorities and after weeks of denial – that 'the novel coronavirus is human-to-human transmissible'. For this he is widely admired and receives countless honours, as well as a Leonid Brezhnev–style gold medal presented personally by Xi Jinping.

During the pandemic Zhong's picture is all over Wuhan. His words appear, laid out like poetry, on posters fixed to shop windows and on walls of high-rise buildings.

Everybody, please cooperate
Medical workers on the front lines
Risk their lives to fight for us
And you

Simply because of boredom
Run about outside
One or two or three people taking a chance
Can undo everything

Not everyone respects the eighty-four-year-old Party veteran. In the eyes of many liberals, Dr Zhong's position and views are dubious. 'He's always been a true Party member,' says Li Xuewen, the independent writer. 'He does whatever the Party wants.' Dr Lin Qingchuan is more direct, to the point of crudity. 'That Zhong Nanshan is just a Party bum-wiper.'

In the spring of 2020, Dr Zhong issues specialist opinions and participates in numerous commercial activities, endorsing products like mineral water, yoghurt and sports drinks. He even promotes a highly controversial traditional Chinese medicine of dubious value: Lianhua Qingwen capsules. These activities engender much criticism and ridicule, though Shao Shengqiang does not object. Shao does not conceal his veneration of Dr Zhong, singing his praises to his circle of friends on social media: 'He can turn tides and prevent the collapse of buildings. He is a peerless counsellor for the state!!!'

Gangcheng's spirits are much lower than his friend's. Every day is pure tedium and every night is painfully long. Over and over, he gazes at pictures of his wife and child, hoping that the return of warm family life will soothe his anxieties. He often doubts himself, doubts the world around him, and doubts the doctor's diagnosis.

On 28 January, spurred on by wishful thinking, he rushes to the Wuhan No. 7 Hospital, hoping to get a nucleic acid test. This is no easy task because the government supplies few tests; even the overworked doctors and nurses can't help themselves. Many patients are forced to wait at home, infecting their own family members. 'Patients with mild symptoms should not go to hospitals,' the government loudly and repeatedly announces. 'Self-isolation at home is the best choice.' It cannot be known how many people die as a result of this policy.

It's a dozen-odd kilometres from Gangcheng's home to the No. 7 Hospital. It is a sunny and cloudless afternoon. Apart from the occasional ambulance, he sees barely a living thing. He finds himself slowing down along the empty streets, not making a sound, as if afraid to disturb something unseen. 'Any loud noise felt discordant,' he says.

On the way he crosses the Yangtze River. Trees and buildings are reflected clearly on each side of the crystalline water, like a scroll painting gradually unrolling as the river water flows quietly by.

Gangcheng drives slowly over the bridge as a group of haggard pedestrians stagger along the footpath. Some are coronavirus patients, others their family members. They are carrying heavy loads in their arms or on their backs.

One old man with white hair pushes a bicycle with one hand and carries a parcel in another hand. He is stooped and puffing, hobbling like a wounded ant.

As Gangcheng watches the old man, he feels a wave of sadness and silently cries.

At the No. 7 Hospital, anxious faces, sorrowful faces, indignant faces bob up and down, struggling in a sea of humanity. Gangcheng cautiously tries to avoid making contact with anyone or anything. Just as he passes the toilets, he hears a loud plonk as a tall youth falls onto a washbasin. Gangcheng shouts for a doctor, then watches as they wheel the youth into the emergency department, as if they have been continuously running under fire on the battlefield. 'It was a scene from an extreme disaster, a picture of utter despair,' says Gangcheng.

There is a six-day wait to book the nucleic acid test.

Those six days are Gangcheng's 'darkest moment', and many months later he still can't conjure up how he managed to hold on. He constantly thinks of death, and how his family will get by after he dies – his old and frail parents, his child not yet two years old.

During this moment Li Qiongli, the local Party secretary, appears on television, portrayed as the hero everyone looks up to. A neighbour sarcastically comments on a residential owners' social media group, 'Never see her, yet somehow she's become an exemplar.' Gangcheng remembers that TV news item but does not want to discuss his impression of it. He does not get angry easily. And even when he is occasionally angry, he deploys a gentle posture and countenance to conceal the anger. 'I am past the age of extremes,' he says, sounding old and worn out.

Upon leaving that darkest moment behind him, Gangcheng is grateful to the whole world. He is grateful for the labours of his parents, he is grateful for the consolation of his close relatives, and he is grateful to Ah Hui for joking with him – 'You're not sick at all, you're just pretending to be sick because you don't want to come home.' Gangcheng knows his wife is helping him 'unload his psychological burdens'. 'She wanted to cheer me up. In fact, she had made preparations just in case I became really sick,' says Gangcheng. 'She had withdrawn our savings.'

Shao Shengqiang is also on Gangcheng's long thank-you list.

Shao's treatment is nearing completion, and he decides to help patients like himself and their anxious relatives by sharing his experience. Gangcheng is one of his first patients. Later Shao reveals to journalists the secret of his 'therapy': 'First, be calm; second, eat well; third, take protective measures.'

Gangcheng does not recall much about 'Mr Shao's three principles' but is grateful for his friend's solicitude. 'Shao Shengqiang is a hyper-zealous type who likes to shout slogans,' he says jokingly, as he imitates Shao's heroic arm-waving pose. '"This disease is not scary. Don't be afraid."'

In a newspaper report titled 'Survivor Shao Shengqiang: twenty-two days of life and death after critical illness', Shao's three principles are explained in detail, especially the first principle: 'There's so much information on the web, but it's fragmented and unsystematic. Some people become more frightened the more they read.' For this reason, you must be calm: 'Don't believe rumours, don't spread rumours. Have a correct understanding of the pandemic.'

These words are exactly the same as the slogans in the newspapers, which have been printed up and plastered on every street in Wuhan and in every neighbourhood. Gangcheng finds them helpful, and from that time on he pays attention to 'mental construction'.

Gangcheng is a film buff who enjoys 'thoughtful and profound' films. However, during the three months of his self-isolation he doesn't watch any movies like that. Instead, he kills time watching superficial movies and even tawdry domestic TV dramas like *The Nanny Man*, *The Bachelor* and *To Be a Better Man*. He takes his friend's advice and pays little attention to the news, and doesn't even look at social media or the 'rubbish that pops up on smartphones'. Like a frightened ostrich burying its head in the sand, he works hard to isolate himself from his hometown's river of tears.

Several months later, he is still avoiding the 'negative news'. He missed many moments that are engraved in the city's mind: the 'gong-beating girl' who banged on an enamel basin in order to seek treatment for her infected mother; the ninety-year-old mother who cared for her infected son in the hospital for four days and four nights, only to receive the news of her son's death.

Gangcheng tries to avoid saying the words 'COVID-19' and 'novel coronavirus'; he says 'the disease' and 'this thing', as if to avoid confronting black magic. He is not the only person observing this taboo. Several months later, when life in Wuhan appears to return to normal, as people happily go shopping and use chopsticks to scoop up steaming hot dry noodles, very few people utter the words 'COVID-19' and 'novel coronavirus'. If someone brings it up, others gently change the subject saying, 'Don't talk about those things. Let's eat!'

Perhaps for this reason, Gangcheng doesn't mind the Chinese government's censorship, and even praises it. 'This is the way our government handles problems. It's ...' He gently rubs his cheek with the back of his hand. 'This approach is understandable.'

*

Shao Shengqiang's WeChat group carries almost no 'negative news'. 'Our nation's system is sound but there are problems with implementation,' says Shao in an April interview. 'I have total trust in the state.' Even when Wuhan is at its most difficult moment, he does not evince a trace of discontent; instead, he deploys exclamation marks and a grandiloquence more suited to speeches from the high podium at a public square.

> *'When the nation faces difficulties, our unity is impregnable!'*
>
> *'Obediently staying at home contributes to the motherland!'*
>
> *'Trust the Party and the state!'*

It is hard to tell if this praise is sincere or a kind of survival skill. In China, every successful businessman must possess this skill. They almost never criticise the government and sometimes argue on the government's behalf, even singing its praises. Shao Shengqiang is highly proficient at this. He never complains – at least not publicly. He is grateful to doctors and nurses; he is grateful to 'the Party and the state'; he is even grateful for the lockdown. Asked in the April interview, 'How do you see the government's deliberate concealment of the pandemic?' Shao confides, 'Some people may be angry at the official concealment, but I'm not.' Looking directly into the eyes of his questioner, he bares his heart: 'After all, I've already died once, am I right?'

In the twelve days Shao stayed in the Red Cross Hospital, he never saw the faces of the doctors and nurses because they wore personal protective clothing and plastic raincoats. Under the PPE, their heads and faces were tightly wrapped in head scarves, protective goggles, and thick masks and visors. To identify themselves, they wrote their names, the names of their hospitals and even their home addresses on their fronts or backs, making them look like soldiers about to set off for a fierce battle.

Shao Shengqiang was looked after by several nurses from Sichuan. They were very fond of this overweight, ebullient patient, calling him 'Brother Fat'. When they weighed him, the scales broke. Shao is not offended and continues to praise these 'nurse sisters', saying they are 'professional, sweet, and enthusiastic'. He even employs an exaggerated Mao Zedong–style phrase: 'We are bound by a profound revolutionary friendship.'

*

On 30 January, Gangcheng rushes into the same hospital. A man in PPE bars his way, saying the hospital is closed and asking him to leave immediately. Gangcheng tells him, 'The doctor told me to come for a re-examination.' The man responds, 'You can't come in for a re-examination. Go ask the neighbourhood committee.'

Gangcheng is baffled. 'Why would I ask the neighbourhood committee? I need to see a doctor.'

The man impatiently waves his hand. 'It doesn't matter what you say, there's no outpatient service now.'

Gangcheng learns that the Red Cross Hospital was undergoing 'rectification', but he doesn't know why. About two weeks later, a news report reveals that the hospital had over four hundred novel coronavirus patients, but its resources were limited, with only enough oxygen for a hundred patients. The report's author mentions that 'some of the patients became more severely ill due to hypoxia'; there is no way to know how many people were affected and how serious their condition really was. In China, not-knowing is not entirely a bad thing, because the people who try to ferret out the truth run into serious trouble. Ignorance is bliss.

Gangcheng instead drives to the Wuhan Central Hospital's Houhu branch, arriving around dusk. Perhaps black motorcycle taxi driver Li is at the door, openly touting for business. In the lobby, Jin Feng weakly nestles in Xia Bangxi's embrace. A little way away in a ward, Dr Li Wenliang is struggling to breathe. A dozen or so hours later he will post that now-infamous reprimand online.

The outpatient building of the Houhu hospital has a rounded corner. On the evening of 30 January, it is crowded with infected patients waiting for treatment in a tiny area with poor ventilation. Gangcheng stands in the midst of the throng for a while but feels the 'environment is appalling'.

'People didn't have any protection awareness. I stood there, doing my best to maintain a distance from people and objects, but others just kept on bumping into me,' says a disgruntled Gangcheng. 'It was damn frightening. I thought I'd rather not get re-examined. I just couldn't stay there any longer.' He flees the 'infected persons market', frantically spraying alcohol sanitiser on his hands and body, and continues on his hazardous journey.

By the time he reaches the Hankou Hospital it is dark. Inside the brightly lit building there is an endless stream of people, not a single smiling face among them. A white car is at the entrance to the hospital, the door open; someone half-seated, half-slumped is receiving an IV infusion, emitting intermittent moans. While standing in line, Gangcheng sees a middle-aged man erupt into a rage at two young nurses. Gangcheng thinks he is making a fuss for no reason.

An hour later, Gangcheng finally gets to see a doctor. The results of the examination make him feel even more dejected. 'I took medicine for six days and not only am I not better, I'm worse.' Nonetheless, the doctor believes his condition is mild and recommends he go home and continue taking medicine.

Gangcheng does not remember how he gets home. It is the most demoralising time of his life.

According to unsubstantiated government figures, forty-three people die of novel coronavirus on this day, of which thirty are from Wuhan. When Gangcheng sees these statistics, he definitely has a lot to think about. For Gangcheng, the Wuhan epidemic is a shock. He believes the Chinese government has become increasingly modernised and able to adapt to society. 'I really didn't think such a situation could emerge,' says a perplexed Gangcheng. 'After suffering such huge losses during SARS, how could the same mistake be made again?'

Gangcheng takes his medicines at the appointed times. The doctor has given him the Russian antiviral Arbidol and the antibiotic norfloxacin, as well as the 'anti-pandemic capsules' promoted by Zhong Nanshan, the thirteen ingredients of which include forsythia (also known as Easter Tree), almond, gypsum and rhubarb. On social media, these traditional medicines are ridiculed: 'Eat too much of this and it'll make you stupid.' In May, Swedish customs prohibits their import because 'there is no research to prove the efficacy of this medicine'. But Gangcheng is not sceptical. He complies with his doctor's instructions: four capsules, three times a day. 'I took medicine like I was eating food, and ate food like I was taking medicine.'

He forces himself to eat. 'I ate three eggs a day and I drank two glasses of milk. Additionally, I was careful I ate fixed portions of vegetables and rice. Even when I had no appetite, I forced myself to eat.' He reads an article saying that a nurse infected with novel coronavirus 'consumed chicken soup like it was medicine' and was subsequently cured. This is an inspiration for Gangcheng. From that day on he cooks a pot of chicken soup every few days. 'I held my nose and gulped it down.'

Gangcheng's relatives and friends call him on the phone, among them Shao Shengqiang. His work colleagues extend helping hands, buying him face masks, alcohol sanitisers, food and even an expensive oximeter. These kind and generous acts warm his heart, but do not improve his health. Ultimately, he must rely only on himself. He becomes even more attentive to 'mental construction' – 'I concentrated on the positive and avoided thinking negative thoughts. I avoided all the rubbish on the mobile phone.'

It might have been the chicken soup or the medicine or perhaps even his mental construction, but gradually Gangcheng gets better. He still suffers bouts of fever, though the durations become shorter.

On 3 February – his daughter's second birthday – Gangcheng gets up and showers, then discovers his temperature is below 36°C. His father visits for lunch and Gangcheng's appetite returns. It's the first time he eats his plate clean. He knows from his discussions with fellow patients that this is a 'clear sign of improvement', though he is careful not to make too much of it because 'there is a lot that is not known about this disease'. And, he observes, 'Physiologically there was improvement but psychologically the torment was far from over.'

Gangcheng chats with his daughter on a video conference for her birthday. His little angel appears to be almost within reach, yet he has no way of embracing her. He is both happy and sad. He sends a rare message to his social media friends which includes several photographs – a family portrait, his daughter pulling a face as she winks. He writes, 'In many years' time you will definitely not remember this special birthday.'

This is also the day Gangcheng goes to the No. 7 Hospital for his first nucleic acid test. The doctor tells him that the results will be telephoned through to him no matter what. But the phone call never comes.

On 5 February, Wuhan's mobile cabin hospitals open. Despite the government's propaganda about this 'grand initiative', Gangcheng is afraid. 'At the time, I felt these mobile cabin hospitals were terrible – just huge bunkhouses without air conditioning despite the cold weather.' He swears profanely. 'How is that different to a concentration camp?' A moment later, that evaluation seems inappropriate, and he mutters, 'It wasn't just me. Everyone thought that.' In Communist Party terminology, Gangcheng and his father belong to the 'patriotic masses'. They support the regime and approve of almost all its actions. But in that time, they reveal that they fear the 'totalitarian prevention and control measures' resemble the actions of the Nazis.

Gangcheng procrastinates, reluctant to go to the hospital to follow up on the test results. 'Picking up the results a day later meant being taken away a day later,' he says. His family and friends agree with him. In the following days, more and more people are 'taken away', initially only people with positive nucleic acid test results, but later a new term, 'the four categories', gains currency: diagnosed patients, their close contacts, suspected infected patients, and those who cannot be ruled out as being infected. All people in these categories are to be 'taken away'.

Just as in the era of Mao Zedong, the term 'four categories' takes on an ominous flavour. Gangcheng and his family worry day and night. One day his father says, 'If you are tested positive, we're finished.'

In Chinese, 'finished' often refers to death or utter defeat.

On 3 February, Secretary Li Qiongli finally telephones Gangcheng. She asks about his medical condition and expresses her concern and condolences. It makes a deep impression on Gangcheng.

Later, he spends several minutes praising her diligence and warm-hearted service to the community: 'In this serious pandemic she's put on the frontlines. How much does she make a month? What sort of situation is she facing? After February third, Secretary Li contacted me every day and helped us buy fifty face masks. I think she's very kind. She sincerely cares for me. By the end of March, people like her had to work to until ten in the evening. Can you imagine what it was like in February?'

In Gangcheng's view, 'the great majority of Wuhan residents' are the same as him, grateful to the neighbourhood committee and the government. But in late February, a woman posts an angry video online, expressing her outrage at her neighbourhood committee's idleness and at the people who praise and defend them. 'We have been mostly helping ourselves, but if we had waited for you, we would have starved to death.' She employs obscure literary allusions, as well as colourful language as she reaches the height of indignation. The video goes viral and is called the 'Wuhan sister-in-law's level ten curses'. Gangcheng is impressed by her literary talent, but he definitely disagrees with her viewpoint.

On 7 February, Ah Hui begins to show symptoms of fatigue, high temperature and severe diarrhoea. Gangcheng becomes extremely anxious, especially because she is in close proximity to his elderly parents and their two-year-old girl. 'That was a difficult time,' he sighs. 'I had just become a little better and now I have to start worrying about her.'

On the same day, the government announces Li Wenliang's death. After dusk, Wuhan citizens open their windows and shout into empty streets in the black of night.

Gangcheng hears the shouting, but indistinctly. 'I was not as overwrought as some people,' says Gangcheng. 'I have always been rational and calm.' He thinks about 'positive things', like the singing of 'Ode to the Motherland', a typical 'red' song that praises China's high mountains, plains and rivers, the five stars on the nation's red flag, Mao Zedong and 'the rising red sun of the east'. Since the 1950s, Chinese people have been born, grown old and died to the sounds of this kind of song. Not far away, one of his neighbours sings:

Our flags are waving in the wind
With the glorious praise of victory
Ode to our gracious motherland
Marching toward prosperity from today

*

Outside Gangcheng's window, the words on the skyscraper opposite are lit up all night; he looks out at them before he goes to sleep. When the whole city 'presses the pause button', almost all manufacturing and business shuts down, and the government turns skyscrapers into signage for slogans. When night-time arrives, the buildings bloom into light, but there is not a soul in sight or sound to be heard; it's like an enormous living room for ghosts. In February, Gangcheng looks out to see, 'Wuhan step on it, China will win,' followed by, 'Salute the white-robed warriors.' In March, as the helpers from all the other provinces withdraw, the slogan becomes, 'Holding their white armour, they return in triumph.' Just before the lockdown is lifted, the skyscraper lights up with, 'Wuhan, how are you?' That sounds like an awkward greeting at a social gathering.

In the mornings, the lights are extinguished but the propaganda slogans do not disappear. On every street, at every intersection, the regime's warnings, advice and threats cannot be missed.

> *'Disobeying the neighbourhood committee's lockdown orders will be severely punished under law!'*
>
> *'Don't chat while eating, don't speak without a mask!'*
>
> *'Obey the Party, always follow the Party!'*
>
> *'Starting now, everyone is a warrior. You are not isolated at home, you are fighting! You may feel bored, but you can bore the virus to extinction!'*

No one objects to these slogans, but no one attaches much importance to them either. People just walk past.

Even the workers who install the slogans don't seem to care. In April, two young men are sticking up some slogans by the East-West Lake Square. One reads: 'When the country is stable, all under heaven is stable; when the people are at ease, the whole world is at peace.' They don't know at whom this slogan is directed and why it is being said. 'Yeah,' says one, bewildered, 'I hadn't really thought about the meaning of what we are sticking up.' The other worker is a little savvier. He cautiously wipes the glue on his hands onto a nearby glass barrier and, without raising his head, says, 'Who cares. The leaders want us to stick 'em up, so we'll stick 'em up.'

From around March 2020, many neighbourhood committees hoist Soviet-style flags printed with the hammer and sickle. It is the flag of the Chinese Communist Party. The sickles represent the peasantry and the hammers the proletariat, indicating the Communist Party is the party of the 'labouring masses'. Some flags are made of paper, others of cotton and silk. They are flown on every corner, giving the whole city a red hue.

Scenes like this are not common in China. According to regulations, hanging a Party flag is a 'solemn and dignified' matter, one that must meet strict guidelines, with a complex application process. In this spring of 2020, however, no one knows how all these blood-red flags appeared in this city of tears, as if it has just been 'liberated'.

The flags are the Party's way of telling the world this is the *Party's* victory over the virus – not the victory of the doctors, the medicines or the tens of millions of obedient citizens. As the slogan everywhere declares: 'Wherever the Party's flag flies, the pandemic dies.'

Beneath the flags and bold slogans, the streets are embroidered with melancholy signs of everyday life. On the front door of a bankrupt beauty salon is a handwritten announcement in faded black scrawl: 'To my friends who bought packages, I'm sorry. I didn't want this to happen but I just couldn't continue.' Not far away, a basket of old celery rests on a shared bicycle. After months of weathering, the leaves are still green but the stalks have rotted.

Outside a shop near the old Wuhan Chongzhen Church hang some wind chimes. Attached below each wind chime are wishes written on small slips of paper: 'I hope in future life is sweet.' 'I hope 2019 passes peacefully and 2020 will be smooth.' As the lockdown is lifted, the shop remains closed and the chimes are covered in grime. The wish slips gently sway and hit the chimes in the evening breeze, like long-forgotten dreams.

*

On 10 February, Gangcheng finally goes to the No. 7 Hospital to collect the nucleic acid test results. It's negative. Although the test result is unreliable, he feels greatly relieved – 'I would not be taken away immediately.' The Wuhan city government announces the number of newly infected patients daily, but Gangcheng reckons he is never included in the statistics. He often says he is a 'suspected suspect case', and Ah Hui – who suffers fourteen days of diarrhoea and low-level fever but never takes any medicine – can be considered a 'suspected, suspected suspect case'.

The No. 7 Hospital is no longer as crowded. Gangcheng undergoes a series of examinations but has to wait a very long time to see a doctor. A nurse tells him that the doctors are busy issuing death certificates. Then the nurse walks over to her colleagues, and, in the cold hospital corridor filled with the smell of disinfectant, the nurses, dressed up like aliens, sing and dance to the beat of happy music while filming a video for Douyin, the Chinese version of TikTok.

Gangcheng remembers that scene well. On one side of the corridor, doctors are signing death certificates; a little further on is a recently deceased person whose corpse has not yet cooled. On the other side, young nurses are singing and dancing. 'Some people will not be able to understand. They may think that someone has just died, so how can they do that? I don't see it that way. I don't think the nurses filming a Douyin video is immoral, I just think ...' He ponders a moment. 'Honestly speaking, I don't really know what I think.'

In the following days, Gangcheng continues his life of an urban hermit, leaving the house rarely, only to take out the rubbish or collect the mail. Even for such short journeys he never forgets to wear a mask and put on gloves, and he always has alcohol sanitiser or disinfectant in his pocket to spray about wherever he goes. Some residents slip out of their homes to stroll around the building, but Gangcheng never joins them. 'I was worried about two things – being taken away and being exposed to the neighbourhood committee. If a neighbour discovered that I had been sick, I would doubtless be taken away. I was afraid it would hurt my family.'

Gangcheng never talks with anyone in the neighbourhood, but he can't deceive the more vigilant neighbours. In the apartment owners' group on WeChat he occasionally sees reports exposing people: 'I heard someone coughing violently.' At times like that, Gangcheng tries hard to suppress his coughing or divide it into segments, first half a cough, then a second half a little later, all the while doing his best to keep the volume down.

One day Shao Shengqiang 'treats' a patient, in tears on the phone, who is already cured of the virus. 'I'm afraid to go out the door,' she says. 'It always feels like the neighbours are talking about me behind my back. They hide when they see me.' Shao sighs dispiritedly: 'How can we avoid this senseless discrimination?' Gangcheng doesn't feel he was discriminated against; he describes this as 'distinctive treatment'. 'Some neighbours had an extreme reaction,' he says, but 'talking about that might not be appropriate.' Sometimes he even reminisces about life under the lockdown. 'That was Wuhan's most harmonious era, when people were extremely harmonious and everyone was very considerate.' He chuckles.

In the days when socialising is not possible, Gangcheng frequently hangs out in WeChat groups with his university classmates, telling them about his medical condition. They express their concern and offer blessings. Yet on 13 February, when Beijing orders the dismissal of Wuhan's Party secretary, none of his classmates respond to his suggestions to chat about the issue. After a few days of silence, Gangcheng discovers that their WeChat group has been blocked.

Such experiences are not unique. During the pandemic, WeChat works closely with the government on information censorship, deploying a workforce who labour like a tiger that never sleeps, staring hard at every single person, every social media group, every item of news. They close thousands of accounts, block family groups, friendship groups, classmate groups, work groups. They never give a reason.

Gangcheng does not remember whether he or a classmate said anything politically sensitive. They all lead comfortable lives, almost never express anger and have few complaints. Their docile attitude is, 'I don't want to stir up trouble.' But sometimes, they will unwittingly cross a line and end up tasting what it means to be 'dealt with by the law'.

'I really don't know why our group was blocked. If I have to guess, I'd say a classmate – his girlfriend works in a street committee – perhaps revealed some internal matters of the street committee.' Gangcheng can't remember what that classmate said; perhaps he doesn't want to remember. Such things do not help with his 'mental construction'.

None of the classmates express any opposition; they just set up a new group. Later they hold a virtual party; Gangcheng goes online early and watches familiar faces pop up one by one. 'Everyone tried to be the first to speak and everyone was laughing. Everyone was so happy,' says Gangcheng. 'Shutting down the WeChat group was only a matter of four or five days, but we all felt, gosh, it's like we were good friends who had been separated for years.'

Their blocked WeChat group contained many years' worth of memories; it was where they had teased each other, argued and exchanged greetings. Gangcheng reviews their chat records from those days, often letting out a laugh.

Then he does something senseless that he finds very satisfying. He posts a question to the blocked group: 'Has the lockdown been lifted today?' He doesn't expect an answer. Like a stubborn child staring through a window at sweets, he repeatedly fires off, 'Has the lockdown been lifted today?'

Gangcheng does not consider this an act of resistance. 'I just feel what I did means something.'

In his view, the blocking of his WeChat group and the lockdown of Wuhan hold the same significance: he is not happy about it, but he is able to accept it. 'I can understand the state's operations and logic for doing so. The West worships so-called freedom, but it won't necessarily work here,' he says quietly. 'I don't feel the West is better than China, you can't generalise like that.

'After experiencing the pandemic,' says Gangcheng, 'the mindset of many Chinese people suffered a huge shock, and their perception and understanding of the West changed greatly. As for the Chinese government's performance, I think it can't be looked at in isolation. You need to look at it in a global context. A comparison of like with like is needed. I think we have to give our country a high score.'

On 22 or 23 February, Gangcheng goes for his second nucleic acid test at the entrance of an isolation hotel. He queues for about forty minutes before walking up to the test counter. A nurse sticks a cotton bud down his throat, jiggles it about, then puts it into a vial.

The cotton bud and a few jiggles cost 180 RMB (A$40). In a city like Wuhan, that's not cheap. In Lin Qingchuan's community hospital, the monthly salary of many nurses is 601 RMB (A$123) – a test like this consumes a week's salary. No one knows who sets the price, and very few people will publicly raise their suspicions. In the days to come, tens of millions of Chinese people are ordered to take – and pay for – the unreliable test. The Chinese government makes billions of RMB from these tests.

Just as Gangcheng is about to leave, a middle-aged woman behind him approaches the test counter. She is a cured patient. It's a cold, windy afternoon and her visage is haggard and anxious. She passes her ID card to the nurse, who registers the number and hands it back to the woman. The woman appears to be afraid of the ID card and instinctively attempts to wipe it with alcohol sanitiser. But she's also afraid of offending the nurse. She freezes momentarily, at a loss.

The nurse glances at her. 'Don't be like that. You've recovered. You have to go on living. That attitude is no good.'

Gangcheng remembers those words. 'You have to go on living,' he says softly, as he recalls so much that has happened. Then he says it again, 'You have to go on living.'

*

Shao Shengqiang talks very little of his difficulties. After the lockdown began, his restaurants had no business and closed down one after another; in Shao's words, it was 'cutting off an arm in order to survive'. No one will cover his 250,000 RMB (A$50,500) medical bill. For several weeks he visits many government offices, but it is all a waste of time. 'I no longer entertain any hope,' he writes on WeChat. 'Living is good enough.'

The disappointment does not affect his love of the government. Every few days, he publicly expresses his gratitude to the Party and government on WeChat: 'Thanks to the Provincial Party Committee Office.' 'Thanks to the United Front Work Department.' 'Thanks to the Women's Federation.'

On 10 March, Xi Jinping visits Wuhan. Shao wastes no time, posting a photo to his social media friends of Xi Jinping wearing a mask and waving. He expresses his loyalty to this great leader in a rhyme: 'In this life I've no regrets a Chinese to be, in future lives it's Chinese for me.'

There's almost nothing about the youthful businessman's character that can be faulted. Looking at his social media posts, he appears to be a morally perfect person. He's patriotic, he loves his family, he loves his subordinates, he even loves total strangers. After his home isolation, he participates in numerous public benefit events. He visits hospitals to distribute baked goods to doctors and nurses – coloured buns in various shapes, little biscuits and tiny cakes. His telephone is always busy; by the end of February he says he has called more than one thousand people to provide his voluntary consultations. 'This is the most meaningful thing I can do now,' he says. 'Ordinary things are the most moving.'

Gangcheng doesn't remember when the cherry blossoms began to bloom, nor did he notice the withered petals swirling in the air, but he is slowly becoming accustomed to the lonely life of isolation. He's even a little joyful. 'I was quite relaxed at that time. Wuhan had the pandemic largely under control, and things were getting better and better.' He wipes his cheek with his wrist. 'The most difficult phase was over.'

In February, he posts to his WeChat friends a passage mimicking Winston Churchill: 'We will fight to the end. We will fight in the hospitals, we will fight in the isolation wards, we will fight with the Hema app ... we shall never surrender.'

'Some people are aware this is Churchill's most famous speech, and some don't know, but all will smile,' says Gangcheng.

'Fresh Hema' is a company that delivers fresh food; during the shortages caused by the lockdown in Wuhan, the company sold several million tonnes of food. Every evening at 9.55 pm – he sets his alarm clock specially to remind him – Gangcheng stops whatever he's doing and rolls up his sleeves to enter battle mode. Five minutes later, Fresh Hema posts new items online. Gangcheng, his classmates and others across the city log on to grab chicken, beef, vegetables and condiments. In just a few minutes, everything is gone.

Gangcheng performs well on this battlefield, but he also suffers defeats. 'Once I wanted to eat beef and selected four catties [two kilos] of tendon as well as Sichuan peppers and other spices. But that day, I bagged the spices but not the beef.

'After the pandemic, many people in Wuhan have a special affection for Fresh Hema,' Gangcheng says passionately. In his middle-class life, to 'grab a Hema' is amusing and even a matter of pride. For Jin Feng the hospital cleaner and Li the black motorcycle taxi driver, Hema has no connection with their lives. They belong to a different Wuhan, an impoverished, humble Wuhan, without Fresh Hema and definitely without beef tendon. It's reasonable to surmise that in this Wuhan, infections and deaths are much higher. They can only look up at the Wuhan of privilege, where people have no concerns about food and few get infected.

Gangcheng's second nucleic acid test is again negative. According to the neighbourhood committee, this means that he can be released from home isolation, though he never receives an actual notification.

Now Wuhan is undergoing a mass screening. Gangcheng calls it a large-scale 'manhunt and purge'. Many suspected infection patients are 'taken away' to mobile cabin hospitals. Although Gangcheng has two negative test results, he is still afraid to go outside, and he's even more afraid to go home to his family. He is often anxious, like a guilty man waiting to be sentenced to jail.

On the evening of 12 March, half an hour before another Hema battle, Gangcheng reads an article on his mobile phone about Dr Li Wenliang. By then, Dr Li's WeChat account has more than 500,000 comments. People pour out their hearts in mourning: 'Dr Li, be happy where you are.' 'Dr Li, I just saw you in a dream, I sobbed silently.' The author of the article quotes many of the comments and is himself deeply moved: 'Before I knew it, I had tears running down my face.' He adds a very sad line: 'Yes, Dr Li, spring has arrived.'

A myriad emotions flood Gangcheng's mind after he finishes reading. He takes pity on Li Wenliang and is saddened by the messages people leave. He weeps, perhaps because he's thinking of his own experience. It really is the most beautiful season in Wuhan. Millions of cherry blossoms drift to the ground like snow. This man who is not so good at expressing his feelings suddenly wants to pour his heart out.

Pent up emotions spur him on to open Li Wenliang's Weibo account and post: 'Dr Li, today is fourteen days after my second negative nucleic acid test.' Tears stream down his cheeks and he sobs sporadically. 'In this case, today is the day my home isolation is formally rescinded.'

'That was the last time during the isolation I had an emotional breakdown. I was already fully cured so I didn't expect I'd have another breakdown, and I didn't expect it would be because of him. I never expected that an article like that would have such a huge impact on me.'

'Fully cured' is not entirely accurate. On 25 March, Gangcheng has his first antibody test; the IgM and IgG antibodies are both detected. This means he still has remnants of the virus in his body.

The government is starting to encourage people to go back to work. Gangcheng is very keen to return to a normal life. Yet he hesitates for several days more. Around the end of March or beginning of April, he again phones Li Qiongli to clarify the rules. Secretary Li's voice is hoarse and she sounds exhausted. 'Get in touch with one of my colleagues,' she says. 'I am busy with burial matters these days.'

The 'burial matters' that keep the neighbourhood committee busy are a sad business, sadder perhaps than the actual burials. Secretary Li's job includes persuading the families of the deceased to hurry up and collect the ashes for burial. Even more important, she must ensure that the 'emotions of the families of the deceased are stable'.

Gangcheng says this telephone call made him feel a little upset 'on two levels. First, the work itself. Second, you can imagine Secretary Li, from the moment of the pandemic's outbreak to this very day, has not had a moment's rest.' He sighs, 'It really is not easy for the people at the grassroots level.'

Several days later, Shao Shengqiang is interviewed in his Eurasian Magpie Bakery. The enterprise employs many staff with hearing loss; in the words of the newspapers 'it is a bakery that speaks in the language of love'. The furnishings and the decorations are very modern. The owner's strong patriotic stance is on display. The bookshelves feature a biography of Mao Zedong and Xi Jinping's *The Governance of China*, as well as Communist Party magazines like *Seeking Truth* and *Party Life*. Some have dog-eared pages, proof they have been read many times.

For the interview, Shao Shengqiang sits upright, displaying his sparkling Communist Youth League medallion. He responds to all questions with alacrity. When speaking of the pandemic, this young man, a Party member of over a decade, nods gently. 'The experience of escaping mortal danger,' he says with a catch in his throat, 'has reinforced my faith in our Party even more.'

On 17 April, Gangcheng has his second antibody test, which confirms he is cured. Wuhan's lockdown is already over but he still does not dare return home to see his family.

As usual, before sleep, he looks at the building across the street. Signs of normal life are starting to appear within the building, but the lights and slogans that stirred the spirits are no more. Gangcheng is disappointed and confused, as if he has lost something but does not know what it is.

'Actually, I have reservations about the ending of the lockdown,' says Gangcheng, 'or rather, I'm a little concerned because I know there are many asymptomatic people as well as rather lax criteria for discharging patients from hospitals. Many people think the lockdown is over and they can go out to shop and dine, so off they rush off. I think we are a long way from that stage.' He falls silent, then adds: 'This pandemic is nature giving humanity a lesson. It is not over, it's far from over.'

He does not return to his family until 25 April. He has not seen his wife and daughter in person for three months – what felt like a lifetime.

He quietly walks into the room and his daughter runs over to him, laughing happily. 'She keeps on laughing, laughing so hard she's squinting. She keeps on saying "Daddy, Daddy". I say I should wash my hands first and she follows me.'

Gangcheng plunges his hands into the water. He feels heat welling up in his chest. He does not want to let his daughter see him cry. 'Don't come close,' he says gently. 'I don't want to splash water on you.'

'Don't worry, Daddy,' his little angel giggles. 'I'll stand a bit further away so I can watch you wash your hands.'

8.

I want a just explanation

On 17 January 2020, a damp winter chill fills Wuhan's streets. But Yang Min is in high spirits, organising a family banquet for her sisters and their children to gather happily together under one roof. They order a table-load of food, open several bottles of wine, and chatter festively. It has not been a good year, but there was now no danger, no tragedy. Yang Min can't complain.

The previous day, Yang Min helped her only daughter, Tian Yuxi, be admitted to hospital. Four months earlier, when Yuxi was diagnosed with breast cancer, Yang Min arranged for her to go to the best hospital, the Wuhan Union Hospital, to have the tumour removed and undergo several sessions of chemotherapy. The operation was successful, and the doctor says there is at least a 98 per cent probability of survival. She now needs only four more sessions of chemotherapy, after which she will be completely clear of cancer.

Yang Min promises to take her daughter on a trip and buy her pretty clothes after Yuxi recuperates a bit more. The most important festival, the Spring Festival, is approaching, and the streets of Wuhan are bustling with people coming and going. The novel coronavirus is silently spreading, though Yang Min and Yuxi are oblivious.

'I saw the news about the police reprimanding Li Wenliang,' says Yang Min. 'They said the internet is not beyond the reach of the law, and that spreading rumours would be punished. I thought, if the government says it's rumours, then it must be false. I have always believed the government.'

For Yang Min, and most Chinese people, believing the government is not simply a good choice, it's the only choice. With a mighty firewall and strict censorship, every newspaper and every television station belongs to the Communist Party and the Chinese government. If they decide to conceal the truth, the people are none the wiser. In that dangerous month of January 2020, all the newspapers and television stations repeat one phrase over and over: there is no danger, there is no danger. Yang Min believes she and her daughter are safe.

Yuxi undergoes a chemotherapy session on 18 January, and the next day she develops a high fever. Yang Min is distressed yet hopeful. She does not know that she and her daughter are in the eye of a raging tempest. In that perilous time, the Wuhan Union Hospital is one of the most dangerous places in China. Concerned to avoid panic, the government has forbidden doctors and nurses from wearing personal protective equipment and prohibits them even more strictly from saying anything about the virus. On that same day, 19 January, an official confirms at a press conference that the novel coronavirus is 'not highly transmissible'. 'The risk is low,' he says. 'It's preventable and controllable.'

Yuxi's high fever does not subside. She has no appetite. 'Even having a sip of water is difficult for her.' Yang Min is pained as though a knife is twisting in her heart. For most parents in China, their child is the most precious thing in their lives, if not the only precious thing. 'She was the hope of the first half of my life, my sustenance for the second half of my life, she was my life.'

Yang Min spends several sleepless nights looking after her daughter. On 23 January a doctor tells her, 'If her fever doesn't recede, your child will be lost.' Yang Min asks the doctor what she should do. The doctor says, 'You have to take her to a specialist fever clinic.'

This is the day of Wuhan's lockdown. If Yang Min knows, she doesn't care. Her daughter is fighting for her life and that is all that matters.

Yang Min rushes Yuxi to the Red Cross Hospital that night. There they encounter a hospital crammed with patients and exhausted doctors and nurses. 'There was nothing there. Nothing to eat, nothing to drink. There wasn't any oxygen for us. Then my daughter had diarrhoea and another high fever.'

Yang Min pauses, tears stream down her face. 'My poor little girl. Chills and then fever. When the chills hit, she said, "Mummy, I'm really cold." I could do nothing. I just embraced her. When the fever came back, she said, "Mummy, I'm really hot." There was still nothing I could do. I wiped her down and helped her bathe.' Yang Min begins to bawl. 'I can't go on, I really can't.'

Yang Min's sorrow and anger frequently disrupt her narrative. She has to wait for her crying to subside to regain the strength to continue, but in a few minutes she is struck by another memory – a particular incident, a small detail, a single sentence – and bursts into tears again.

On 24 January, Yang Min wheels Yuxi to a room for a CT scan. Both of Yuxi's lungs are covered with white opacities. The doctors confirm Yuxi is infected with the novel coronavirus. She is critically ill, but the hospital can provide no treatment. Like all the other hospitals in Wuhan at the time, the Red Cross Hospital has almost completely run out of medicine and supplies. Yang Min has no choice but to drag her febrile daughter to another hospital.

Cold rain is sheeting down as CCTV broadcasts the New Year's Gala to the entire world. Celebrities sing and dance in praise of the Communist Party and rejoice in China's new era of greatness. Twelve hundred kilometres away, Wuhan is deathly silent. A solitary car traverses the deserted, rain-swept city then stops at the entrance of the Wuhan Jinyintan Hospital.

By now Yuxi is unable to walk. She breathes heavily, while her mother struggles to hold her waist and labours to heave her into the hospital. On TV, the gala program reaches a climax. 'Shout it, shout it loudly,' sings Jackie Chan on the glittering stage. 'Does my country look sick?'

At that very moment, the Wuhan Jinyintan Hospital might be the most deadly place in the world. Chinese media call it 'ground zero of ground zero'. Heavily infected people arriving from all over the city crowd every floor and every room, feverish and coughing. Many of the doctors and nurses, also infected with the virus, weave in and out to the sound of wails and groans. Like sailors on a sinking ship watching passengers bobbing about in icy waters, they are powerless to save others and unable to help themselves.

This New Year's Eve is like a nightmare. The winter rain patters down as Yang Min shivers in the hospital entrance, not allowed to go inside with her daughter. 'The doctor told me "This is a disaster zone. Relatives are not allowed to act as carers."'

Her home is fourteen kilometres from the hospital. She is cold, hungry and exhausted, but is unable to find a taxi or a place to stay. In the end she phones her husband – Old Tian, as she affectionately calls him.

Mr Tian searches everywhere for help, hoping to borrow a car. After three hours he finally finds a generous friend. He walks several kilometres in the rain to his friend's home to pick up the key, then drives to the Jinyintan Hospital. By now it is almost midnight, and the CCTV gala compere is enthusiastically praising the great achievements of China's economy and the victory of 'targeted poverty alleviation'. Then the New Year bell rings, everyone stands up and joyfully cheers: Happy New Year!

Yang Min is sprawled out on the damp floor outside the Jinyintan Hospital. 'I felt I was dying.'

Yuxi, left behind in the hospital, lies helpless on a narrow cot, too weak to turn on her side. She is not receiving any treatment. She sends a stream of text messages to her mother. 'Cold.' 'Aching joints.' 'Can't breathe.' She is constantly coughing, can't eat and is lying in her own excrement. 'There's not a dry spot.' 'It's wet.' 'It's unbearable.' A nurse who sees her soiled bed scolds her. 'Are you playing with faeces?'

'My daughter is shy. If a nurse shouts at her, she won't say a peep,' says Yang Min tearfully. 'She's too scared to press the call button and dares only tell me.'

Finally back at home, Yang Min gazes at a picture her daughter sent and watches her video messages.

Hearing the sound of her daughter's laboured breathing is heartbreaking.

Yang Min is uncertain about when she herself became infected. She frequently coughs and has a low fever. But over the next few days there is nothing she can do other than observe from a distance and try to comfort her. 'Hang in there,' she texts. 'Be strong.' 'Mum loves you.'

At 10 am on 28 January, Yuxi tells her mother on WeChat, 'I vomited blood again.' She sends a photo of her hands, the fingertips all black.

The next day a doctor calls to say Yuxi's condition is 'not very good'. In the Wuhan dialect, that means 'critically ill'.

'Nothing else mattered; I rushed to the hospital,' says Yang Min.

Her husband delivers her to the Jinyintan Hospital, where she slips past security and sneaks into Yuxi's ward. Soon, several nurses and security guards approach. 'They wanted me to leave. I said to them, "If you try to kick me out, just let me die. My daughter is my life. You are doing nothing for her so you can't stop me looking after her."' Yang Min tells them she will 'risk her life to stay here'.

A man shouts a command for the security officers to drag her away. Yang Min is desperate and furious. She shouts, 'If you do this to me, I'll jump off the roof so you can watch me die!'

The man admonishes her sternly. 'It's for your own good,' he says. 'If you get sick, we can't be held responsible.'

Yang Min raises her head. 'I don't need you to be responsible.'

Over the next seventy-two hours, Yang Min never has more than ten minutes' sleep. The hospital has brought an iron-frame bed, but she hardly has a chance to lie down. Yuxi is becoming sicker, despite now being on a ventilator. She is still vomiting blood and probably realises that her time is almost up. She calls for her mother incessantly. 'She just didn't let me rest. She kept on saying she was in pain, uncomfortable, and asked me to caress her here and then stroke her there,' says Yang Min, choking up. 'I said, "Let Mum rest a little so I can better look after you." But no. She just wouldn't let me sleep.'

Yang Min keeps remembering her precious daughter squirming on the hospital bed, struggling to open her mouth, gasping for breath. 'Like a fish just scooped out of the water,' says Yang Min.

Yuxi has a dream. After she wakes up, she holds Yang Min's hand. 'Mummy, I saw you in my dream, but I couldn't find you,' she whimpers. 'Mummy, I'm afraid of not being able to see you.'

Yang Min bawls. 'I'll never forget that sentence: "I couldn't find you in my dream."'

At noon on 1 February, Yuxi is wheeled into ICU. She keeps her yearning eyes on Yang Min, like an injured lamb. 'I sensed she was begging me,' says Yang Min. But she doesn't know what her daughter is begging for.

About a minute later, Yang Min passes out. 'I had been relying solely on mental strength to hold myself together. That fell apart as soon as my daughter was wheeled into ICU. I collapsed.'

*

Yang Min's summary of her own life is simple: 'Born in 1970, joined the workforce in 1987, married in 1992, gave birth to a daughter in 1995.' Then she jumps straight to how she threw herself into bringing up her daughter.

Yang Min's husband, Mr Tian, is a Party member and police officer. After graduating from high school, Yang Min 'inherited' her father's job at a state-run railway company. They are not poor, but they are not rich either. 'I went to work, came home from work, and scrimped on food to raise my child,' says Yang Min. 'That's what it was like in those days. Everything for the child because the child is everything.'

In China under Communist Party rule, the word 'children' for many years lost its plural sense. It actually referred to 'only child'. Yang Min recalls seeing a short film when she was young called *The Guerrillas Who Exceeded the Birth Quota*. This was the cruellest time of family planning in China; every year countless pregnancies were forcibly terminated, and countless families were driven to penury by fines for unauthorised births. The short film was broadcast on national TV and every Chinese citizen knows the story. A peasant couple, trying to avoid being fined for having a child, runs from the southernmost tip of China in Hainan island to Turpan in the north-west, then from the central mountain ranges to the seaside in the east – a journey of more than 10,000 kilometres. The film ridicules their ragged appearance, their poverty and their ignorance, as well as their vagrant life. It was all to teach millions of Chinese that family planning is not only correct, but also wise and important, just like the Communist Party behind the policy.

Yuxi was born in that era. Yang Min still remembers the ubiquitous propaganda slogan: 'One child is good; the government will take care of the elderly.'

'I've always obeyed the law and responded to government appeals,' she says. 'Soon after my child was born, I received the single child certificate and got an intrauterine device.' In government propaganda, the majority of women 'voluntarily' had IUDs inserted, but Yang Min knows that is not true. 'They blackmailed you over work. If I had a second child, Old Tian and I would be fired,' she explains. 'Without work, how can you live?'

From Yuxi's third birthday, Yang Min took her to an endless stream of classes – violin, Chinese chess, calligraphy, Latin dance ... Her grades were always strong and she reached a professional level on the violin, appearing on stage many times.

Children who are not from privileged families have to grow up quickly. Yuxi was well aware of her parent's travails, and frequently said she would look after them in their old age.

Yang Min has barely noticed that her daughter has grown up. She takes an interest in what her daughter wears, what she eats, and what sort of boyfriends she has. She's still like a mother hen taking care of a chick, using affectionate names like 'sweetie', 'baby' and 'darling little Yu'.

In 2012, Yuxi took the university entrance examination and chose bioengineering; after she graduated in 2016, she went to work in Shenzhen, across the river from Hong Kong. Yang Min didn't approve of her daughter's career choice; although the pay would be good, it's hard work, and what she saw as a man's specialty. Yuxi replied: 'Mummy, I want to make a lot of money so that when you get sick, I won't have to sit crying outside the operating theatre.'

*

On 2 February, the day after Yuxi is admitted to the ICU, Yang Min struggles to send her daughter a text message: 'Persevere. You must hang in there, Sweetie. Mummy loves you.' Yang Min then passes out again.

After several hours of emergency treatment, she slowly regains consciousness. Then with trembling hands she types out another message: 'Did you receive the message saying Mummy loves you? Mummy's waiting for you, but of course you know that.'

Yang Min is treated in the Jinyintan Hospital for thirty-two days. 'My lungs felt like they were full of broken glass. Each breath took all my energy.' Even at her sickest, she's thinking about what she can do for her daughter. 'I kept on telling myself, I must get treated to get better as soon as possible so that I'll have the energy to look after her.'

On 11 February, Yang Min's condition stabilises. She sends another message to Yuxi: 'Sweetheart, perseverance means victory. Mummy will definitely be by your side … you have to persevere, Mummy is persevering.'

Yang Min senses something out of the ordinary: on calls, Mr Tian becomes evasive when he talks about their daughter, and the doctors and nurses avert their eyes. She forces herself to avoid thinking about it. 'I became scared when my phone rang. Whenever it vibrated my heart skipped a beat. I wouldn't answer any calls from relatives.' In video messages, Mr Tian appears defeated and old, but he tells his wife, 'Just concentrate on recovering. Don't worry, no news is the best news.'

Someone tells Yang Min that the blood of cured patients can help other critically ill patients. This gives her hope. 'I forced myself to sit up, determined to get well fast so I could have my blood drawn to save my daughter.' She is still sending messages to Yuxi. 'Get well soon.' 'Persevere, I want to be able to chat with you.'

Yang Min gets up on 19 February and sends a WeChat message to Yuxi to tell her she is not yet able to leave the hospital. Although the CT scan shows no improvement, she feels much better. 'It'll still take about seven or eight days. Then I'll be able to take care of you. Keep on fighting, Sweetie.'

Yuxi has been dead for many days. She spent the final moments of her life on 6 February alone in intensive care at the Jinyintan Hospital, then she was taken to a crematorium and reduced to ashes. No one knows what Yuxi saw or said before dying, or how she travelled that sad and arduous path. Twelve days later, her uncle, Mr Tian's older brother, also succumbs to the virus on a hospital bed.

Yang Min knows nothing of this.

After she sends the 'Keep on fighting, Sweetie' message, Yang Min phones her husband to get him to ask the doctors if they can draw some of her blood to treat Yuxi. At first Mr Tian continues to encourage her to concentrate on getting well, but then all of a sudden he flares up and angrily berates Yang Min: 'You aren't better yet, how could your blood be useful?'

Mr Tian's reaction is not like him. 'Something felt wrong.' Rising from her sickbed, Yang Min uses her mobile phone to call the hospital where she is currently being treated. She asks a doctor, 'Tian Yuxi is my daughter, what's her condition? Would it be possible to draw some of my blood to treat her infection?'

The doctor checks the records and responds in an emotionless voice, 'Tian Yuxi? No such person here.'

Yang Min trembles. She calls Mr Tian again and impatiently demands, 'What's going on with our daughter? Tell me now.'

At the other end, Mr Tian breaks down. 'Your daughter departed on the sixth. And my older brother, he left on the eighteenth.' Fifty years old, Mr Tian is wailing loudly. 'If you had waited any longer to ask, I would have lost it. And every day I still have to face you. Do you know how I've been surviving these days?'

Yang Min freezes for a long time. She gradually becomes aware of her hands and feet. Mr Tian is still crying at the other end of the line. She slowly turns around and step by step returns to the bed. She sits down. 'Even my nose and ears were throbbing.' Then she throws down her mobile phone and begins to howl.

Yang Min does not remember how the next few days passed. 'It was a blur, I was in a muddle.' She couldn't eat and refused to answer the phone. She would cry at any time.

At 5.40 pm on 29 February, Yang Min sent another message to Yuxi: 'You just abandon me like that? Is that how you treat your mother?'

She looks at her phone through her misted-up eyes and waits, as if Yuxi will reply from another world. Some three hours later she commands a daughter who is no longer among the living: 'Come home tonight, let me see you again.'

'I didn't even get to see her one last time,' says Yang Min. 'If I'd known earlier, I wouldn't have let her go to the ICU, I would have stayed with her, I would have ...'

Her daughter's death crushes Yang Min. She lies in bed flipping through photos of her daughter and listening to her voice messages. The more she looks, the more she cries. She describes her condition at that time as numb as a yam. She frantically searches the internet for information about 'returning from the grave' and 'rebirthing' in the hope of being able to see her precious daughter again, no matter how faint the chance. 'Just one sight would be enough, just a glimpse.'

On 4 March, the hospital announces that Yang Min is cured and must move to an isolation facility at Hubei University. She refuses to go, grabbing hold of the bed railing and pleading with the doctors to let her stay a few more days. The hospital is an uncomfortable place, but she won't leave because this is where her daughter died. The ward and the narrow hospital bed are her last refuge; as long as she stays there, she will be far from the outside world, the world in which her daughter no longer resides.

Eventually, Yang Min goes into isolation in the Hubei University dormitory. She's there for fourteen days and after that has to isolate herself at home for a further fourteen days. During that period the cherry blossoms have silently bloomed and withered. She is always crying. 'I almost went crazy twice. They made me telephone a psychologist. I cried for three hours,' she recalls. 'The psychologist cried with me.'

Yang Min longs to see her daughter in her dreams, but Yuxi never comes. Someone tells her that a stick of incense is necessary to see a spirit in one's dreams. She burns incense every night, but still nothing.

Traditional Chinese funerary rites last forty-nine days, seven times seven days, after a person dies. Then relatives and friends hold a memorial service and give their blessings so the deceased can make it to the next world or reincarnate. But this spring, hardly anyone is able to offer sacrifices to the lonely ghosts of the departed. Yang Min is worried about Yuxi's life in the next world. 'She died in the ICU and I suppose she was not wearing any clothes.' She begins to cry again. 'When she arrives in the next world, she'll be naked.'

On 18 March, Yang Min returns home. Yuxi has been dead for forty-one days. Yang Min looks around, feeling lost. It is as if her daughter is close by. Her bracelet is still on the table, her dress is still on the clothes rack, but she's not there.

Yang Min sets up a simple altar for the forty-second day after her daughter's passing – the sixth seven-day period. Seeing her daughter's photo, a lifetime of grievance and pain floods her mind, and she collapses to the ground, possessed by tears.

That night, Yang Min's wish to see her daughter is fulfilled. Yuxi appears in a dream. She walks into the room, looks at her mother, and scratches at the door of the closet. Yang Min knows it is not real, yet she dares not make a sound for fear of frightening off that timid soul. Yuxi walks slowly to the bed, lifts the blanket and lies next to Yang Min, just as she did when she was a timorous high school student, when mother and daughter lay head to head, chattering endlessly about Yuxi's headaches, her friends, about every place she's ever been.

Suddenly, Yang Min wakes up, gazing into the darkness in a daze. It is a long time before she remembers her daughter is dead. She cries into the boundless silence.

*

In the spring of 2019, Yang Min and Yuxi travelled to Thailand. On the tour bus they sang China's national anthem, the 'March of the Volunteers', with their fellow travellers. 'Arise, ye who refuse to be slaves! With our flesh and blood, let us build a new Great Wall!' After seventy years of Communist Party rule, the anthem and the Party are firmly bound together. When Yang Min sings this song in a foreign land, her intention is clear – she loves her country and she gives her allegiance to the Chinese Communist Party.

Yang Min never hides her record of 'love the Party, love the country'. Her entire life she has answered the state's appeals, never for a moment doubting the Communist Party's grandiose propaganda and even cheering it on. On 1 October 2019, the seventy-year anniversary of the Communist Party coming to power, Xi Jinping presided over a military parade of unprecedented scale at Tiananmen Square. Yang Min watched the TV broadcast with so much pride that tears streamed down her cheeks. She forgot about the infamous massacre that took place on the same spot thirty years earlier. In her social media group, she was full of praise for the formidable military might on display: 'Awesome, my country, I am proud of you!' Meanwhile, the citizens of Hong Kong were resisting the national security law with mass demonstrations. Yang Min denounced these 'Hong Kong independence elements' attempting to split the nation, even describing their actions as 'heinous'.

After Yuxi died, Yang Min is forced to deal with the regime at close quarters. Gradually she sees through words like 'wise', 'great' and 'correct', as if awakening from a dream. 'I too am Chinese. I have been obeying the Party, I have been obeying the government, I followed your policies to have only one daughter, but due to your concealment of the truth, my daughter died in vain. What is to become of me in later life? Is my life worth nothing? Only later did I know that it was all false.'

Yang Min comes to feel that Yuxi has been sacrificed for no purpose. 'If the government had announced the pandemic a little earlier, I would not have sent her to the hospital. If the hospital had reminded me to pay attention to protection, my daughter would not have died. My child suffered so much,' she sobs. 'She survived a major operation but couldn't be saved – whose fault is that? Do I get an explanation? Can I receive a just explanation?'

Anger and grief do not make her irrational. When some journalists see her social media posts and ask to interview her, she declines. She wants to follow 'normal procedure' through the proper channels. In the middle of March, she makes a verbal complaint to the neighbourhood committee – the lowest level of the Party and government – but receives no response. Early in April, after the lockdown is lifted, she writes a formal complaint, again following the 'normal procedure' – first presenting the materials to the neighbourhood committee, which should then pass them on to the district, the city, the province ... No one knows how far her complaint will go. 'I trusted that my Party and my government would give me justice,' she writes on Weibo.

On 7 April, the neighbourhood committee invites her to a meeting. A Party secretary surnamed Jin expresses condolences and sympathy, then asks her what she wants. Yang Min produces her complaint materials and says she wants an investigation into 'the crimes against humanity' of the official who covered up the pandemic, and compensation for her economic and emotional losses.

Secretary Jin does not see it the same way. He clears his throat, smiles, then says he does not think the government had covered it up, because as early as 31 December 2019 the government announced online there was an epidemic.

This enrages Yang Min. As she later put it on Weibo: 'I finally saw what shameless looks like, what no sense of shame means.' She defies Secretary Jin. 'If you made that announcement, why were you rebutting rumours on TV? Why was Li Wenliang reprimanded? Isn't that like slapping yourself in the face? You call that being responsible?'

These acerbic words go straight to the point, but Secretary Jin is unmoved. He chuckles, fobbing her off: 'This is perhaps a case of the information we received being, um, different.'

There is an infamous catchphrase in communist China: 'Stability trumps everything.' Regardless of the size of the disaster or the number of dead, the newspapers and the television news will always relay the same words: 'The family members of the deceased are emotionally stable.'

These words cover over uncountable deaths, blood and tears, providing no peace for grieving families, and none for their deceased loved ones.

After the neighbourhood committee meeting, the government sends a mediator to talk to Yang Min. Mr Jiang is a little over sixty and was previously a teacher. He is not officially a government employee, but after this disaster many people like Mr Jiang appear in Wuhan. They work closely with the government to carry out a sinister war of attrition against family members of the deceased like Yang Min.

From their first meeting, Mr Jiang exhibits masterful communication skills. He calls Yang Min 'Little Min' and tells her to call him 'Elder Brother'. They engage in small talk for quite a while before slowly approaching the topic at hand. Elder Brother Jiang hopes that Little Min will abide by normal procedures in her complaint. 'Taking the matter further up is alright, taking the litigation approach is also acceptable, but you must not be interviewed by foreign media,' he tells Yang Min. 'You are Chinese, Little Min, and you must be vigilant against hostile anti-China forces. Don't let them use you.'

Yang Min uses a rather sad moniker on Weibo, 'The Crying Dead Soul', to write of her own misery, of her memories of Yuxi and her sharply worded complaints: 'Without a just explanation, the dead will not agree, so of course the living will be even less able to accept.'

Unsurprisingly, she soon receives a phone call from the police. They are quite gentle and merely remind her not to 'publish sensitive remarks online' because they 'would have a negative influence on the country'.

Yang Min sees their point of view. By this time the virus has spread around the world, while the Chinese government is energetically boasting about its own victory over the virus, encouraging every country to learn from China's experience. For most of Yang Min's life, foreign media has been portrayed as sinister and evil, something to avoid, like wild beasts. 'I have always believed "the meat falls apart as it stews, and it stays in the pot". I was born under the red flag, I grew up under the red flag, and there is no need to tell foreigners about Chinese matters. As long as my country gives me justice, I will not make so much fuss that the whole world knows about it.'

On 10 April several relatives go to the mortuary to collect Yuxi's ashes. Yang Min takes to Weibo, recounting Yuxi's cheerful and vivacious appearance and their familiar conversations, now heartbreaking to recall: 'Mummy, let's go out to eat hot pot.' 'Mummy, I bought you a mobile phone cover.' 'Mummy, remember to drink water.' Tears roll down Yang Min's face as she writes, 'All this could have been avoided. Who can I tell it to? Bring my daughter back!'

The Weibo post elicits two thousand comments. Some remind her not to write things that do not correspond with mainstream socialist values, that all things should take the nation's interests into consideration. Some send harsh warnings – the government has done such a good job, what she is writing is handing a knife to the foreign anti-China forces! Some are cruel: don't further burden your dead daughter with more sins.

Although she has no proof, Yang Min is certain these people have been mobilised by the government. Everyone knows about the 'fifty centers' whom the government pays to post pro-government comments and attack dissidents – high school students, retired civil servants, even jailbirds, who can earn merit and reduce their sentences. For each post they are said to receive 0.5 RMB: fifty cents. Yang Min is outraged. 'I write on Weibo about my grievances, my pain,' she exclaims, 'yet they send the fifty centers to vilify me, to say I don't understand the country. Of course I sympathise with my country but does my country sympathise with me?'

A new nightmare begins. Yang Min soon discovers that the blood-stained words she posts on social media either disappear or are reset to 'only viewable by the author'. And the malicious taunting and cursing escalates. 'Traitor! Retard! Get the hell out of China!' At the same time, the 'consolation' phone calls from the police and officials become more frequent and more impatient. The officials she meets no longer smile. 'Don't think what you've been doing is going unnoticed,' one says menacingly. 'State security knows all about you.'

It takes time for Yang Min to become accustomed to her new status. She's no longer a docile subject who 'obeys the Party and reassures the Party'. She's now a suspicious and destabilising element. Still, wherever she goes, she always says emphatically, 'I do not want to overthrow the Party, nor do I want to split the country. I simply want justice.'

This kind of 'gentle resistance' doesn't move the government. The government excels at employing cruel methods on people who dare to voice different opinions and is rarely moved by moderate and restrained words. It's clear about what trouble means – trouble is *trouble*.

After the lockdown is lifted, Wuhan's weather becomes warmer, but Yang Min's world grows colder. Only Elder Brother Jiang remains kind to her. He visits and phones almost every day. Apart from reminding her not to 'be used by anti-China forces', he appears to be willing to help her solve her problems. 'Fill in the form, claim the 20,000 RMB [A$4100],' he urges Yang Min.

Elder Brother Jiang is referring to Yuxi's hospital expenses. Although the government has promised that 'all medical fees of novel coronavirus patients will be covered', Yang Min had paid over 20,000 RMB. Over the course of a month Elder Brother Jiang rushes about helping Yang Min apply for the money to be reimbursed but he fails. There is always an excuse – wrong procedure, missing materials, the person in charge is out. He often mentions 'the Party and government's kindness', but in practice the kindness is elusive.

'Go bury your daughter's ashes, then you will get the money,' Elder Brother Jiang tells Yang Min. 'It's for your own good.' The government is afraid that the families will carry funeral caskets onto the streets. It's a dangerous image, sufficient to ruin the regime's strenuous whitewashing.

Furious, Yang Min retorts, 'That suggestion is an insult to me! You really think that tiny bit of money will buy my daughter?'

As for her complaint, it does not travel as far as she'd hoped. At the end of April, Yang Min contacts an official surnamed Ke and asks him why she has not received an answer. Director Ke tells her, 'Right now we are in the process of helping you apply for a charitable donation.'

Yang Min says, 'I want justice!'

Director Ke replies, 'Your daughter was infected in hospital. Have you considered suing the hospital?' Then she tells Yang Min, 'We are not authorised to reply to your questions or solve your problem. We can only forward to a higher level.' Once again, Yang Min is instructed to go through 'normal procedures'.

Yang Min finally comes to a realisation. There is no such thing as normal procedures. It is all a dead end.

All those people – Secretary Jin, Elder Brother Jiang, Director Ke, the police, the fifty centers – are roadblocks on her path. They will never give her justice, they never even intended to give her justice.

'Now I don't think about the meat falling apart as it stews and staying in the pot,' Yang Min declares at the end of April. 'Starting from now, I will share my grievance with every person I see, regardless of who hears, and regardless of their reaction. If I don't get justice for my daughter, then I'm unworthy of being her mother.'

*

'When I woke up today my tears had saturated my pillow … Daughter, can you feel Mummy's tears and sense my longing for you? Are you missing your mum over there?'

Yang Min types those words in a Weibo post on 10 May. It is Mother's Day. When Yuxi was alive, she'd buy a large bunch of carnations for Yang Min on this day every year. When Yang Min accepted the gift, she always smilingly grumbled that her daughter was squandering money, but on Mother's Day 2020 all Yang Min feels is pain and rage.

'I can't take any more, I can't live well, I can't die. Every day I wake up tormented. One day I had a fight with my husband. He wanted me to lead a normal life,' says Yang Min, deeply hurt. 'But what is a normal life? Can my life ever be normal again?'

She attempts suicide. Mr Tian embraces her tightly, dragging her away from the window. He tries his best to console his wife, but after a few sentences he too begins weeping. Then they cry together.

It's hard to tell how many people's lives in Wuhan have been destroyed by the catastrophe. Every night from late August to early September in 2020, a strange smell lingers in the air. It is the season of the Ghost Festival, a time to worship deceased relatives. Residents come out in small groups. Many are children and elderly people. They draw circles on the ground and burn joss paper as offerings to the dead.

A blogger observes: 'In the past few days, people holding commemoration rituals can be seen everywhere. During evening strolls, I saw one group after another. There was fire everywhere and ash was in the air. Wherever I walked, I could smell the ash.' The post attracts many comments online.

'After living in Wuhan for so many years, for the first time I see so many people burning joss paper.'

'On footpaths there are many circles. There must be a lot of longing in Wuhan this year.'

'Time flies but pain will never be far away. It is as despondent as this city. But carrying on is the only choice.'

This is also how Yang Min feels – furious, despondent, but with no choice but to carry on. She tries some different tacks. She consults a fortune teller, she seeks out monks, she even considers adopting an orphan to start over again. But that would be tantamount to abandoning her beloved daughter, causing her endless sorrow and regret, in this life and the next. She tries to tell herself that it is all down to fate; perhaps over many previous lives she accumulated too much debt to her daughter, so in this life she has to repay it with her broken heart and her tears.

It's no use. She cannot accept such a fate, let alone sympathise with the government's indifference and cruelty. She grows angrier by the day; perhaps the rage helps her live on, like a light at the end of a gloomy tunnel, leading her to move forward, which is not as bad as dying of despair.

'My child has died,' she tells Mr Tian's sister-in-law, Zhang Yanping, whose husband had passed away on 18 February. 'I no longer have anything to look forward to, so I have to keep on fighting.' Yanping also despises the government's cover-ups, but she is not as tough and stubborn as Yang Min. During the interview she speaks softly, repeatedly wiping her tears. Occasionally she tells Yang Min, 'Don't talk about that,' or, 'Don't think about that.'

Yang Min mentions their mother-in-law, Yuxi's octogenarian grandmother. 'I still haven't been able to tell her. She brought up my daughter. If she were to ask me, what could I say?'

Yanping sounds as if she is choking. 'Stop, please,' she pleads. 'She phoned a few days ago asking how her son was. I said, "He's good, he's good, he's good ..."' She raises her head and sobs loudly. 'What else can I say?'

As Yang Min vows to seek justice for her daughter, Yanping too hopes to get some justice for her husband. But she knows how difficult such a path would be. 'I was apprehensive,' she says hesitantly, 'because I have a child.' She looks at Yang Min helplessly and repeats, 'I have a child.'

They constantly feel anxious. When walking they feel they are being followed. On WeChat they studiously avoid 'sensitive words'. During this interview, they look around the room. Yang Min says, 'Can we be monitored here?' Yanping mutters, 'If they overhear ...' They glance at each other. Yang Min stands up and says, as if speaking to an invisible demon, 'Anyway, we don't want to overthrow the Party and we don't want to split the nation. We simply want justice.'

Yang Min knows the price of resistance. She says she doesn't care about the abuse and slanders from the fifty centers. 'I can ignore them.' She is not afraid of the officials' threats and the police reprimands. She is not afraid, either, of being classified as a 'mental patient'. 'I've already thought it through.' As for being arrested and sentenced, she hesitates. 'Well, of course I don't want that.' She is quiet for a moment. 'But I'm not afraid.' This not entirely true. It is more like Yang Min's 'whistling at night'. When she decided to embark on the arduous path of seeking justice, she did not know what was waiting for her in the dark and where the path might lead her to. To overcome her anxiety, she tells herself again and again: I'm not afraid, I'm not afraid.

On 11 May, she walks down the street carrying a portrait of her daughter. The lockdown has been lifted for more than a month; the citizenry is walking about, shopping, playing in the park, as though life has returned to normal. Yang Min walks into their midst wearing a face mask and a blue sun visor, a white shirt and a pair of blue denim jeans. On her front and back hang homemade cardboard placards. On the front is written, 'The government covered up the truth about the pandemic – Bring my daughter back.' On the back is just one large word in red: 'Injustice.'

She walks up to the compound of the Communist Party's Wuhan committee, sits down in front of a bed of four seasons begonias in flower, and places the portrait of Yuxi and the 'Bring my daughter back' placard on the ground in front of her. She then begins to tell her story to passers-by.

It's an extremely dangerous act. Soon, four men rush out of the building's entrance. One policeman goes to where she is sitting. Another grabs her placard. 'You must follow normal procedures,' he says. An official dressed in black repeatedly waves and commands, 'You go over there.'

Yang Min springs up and snatches the placard from the policeman's hands. 'You cannot take my things. This is my private property.' She turns to the official. 'Why should I go over there? Why?'

Yang Min is predestined to lose this battle. After a brief struggle, several more policemen emerge from the main entrance and force her into a small anteroom. The scene that follows is not difficult to imagine. She is reprimanded, mocked, and her private property is confiscated. After about two hours she is released, but she still refuses to leave. She sits on the ground and cries until she is hoarse, attracting passers-by who stand around her watching. The officials and the police are obliged to carry out their duties; they berate her repeatedly and try to chase her away. Yang Min will not move. She shouts to the passers-by, 'Why did the government cover up the epidemic? Several thousand people died. Why won't the government take responsibility?'

A woman comes over to chat. Yang Min tells her of Yuxi's suffering and once again begins to wail. 'Heavens, open your eyes. Does this world still have any justice?'

Before citizen journalist Zhang Zhan was arrested, she posted numerous videos about Yang Min. 'I support Yang Min's actions,' she says in a YouTube video. 'I am prepared to stand with her.'

The day after Yang Min's walk to the committee building, she and Zhang Zhan arranged to meet back at the building's entrance. Zhang Zhan waits nearly an hour, but she sees no trace of Yang Min. She later learns of Yang Min's 'house arrest'. The government had dispatched several guards to Yang Min's neighbourhood, prohibiting strangers from entering her home and Yang Min from leaving. Yang Min stood behind the firmly shut cast-iron gate, holding onto its bars, still dressed in her denim jeans, sun visor and white shirt, on which is written the word 'Injustice'.

On that day's video, Zhang Zhan says this kind of house arrest is unacceptable. 'I am greatly saddened … I hope the government will repent.' She even reads a passage from the Bible to Yang Min, but it is not much help. Zhang Zhan admits to being dispirited. 'I don't know how to console her.'

This is probably one of the reasons Zhang Zhan is arrested. Several days later, the police telephone Yang Min asking how she knows Zhang Zhan and what they have talked about. Yang Min answers honestly: 'I know her. I asked her to read the Bible to me.' The police are obviously displeased by her answer.

After several more days, someone who claims to be

a Japanese journalist telephones to say Zhang Zhan has been released and asks Yang Min for a comment. Yang Min says: if she's out, then get her to phone me. The 'Japanese journalist' replies that it is not convenient for Zhang Zhan to make a phone call. Yang Min asks, 'What's not convenient about making a phone call?'

'Now I'm reluctant to be interviewed by journalists because I can't tell who is real and who isn't,' Yang Min tells a group of her friends on Signal, an encrypted app.

Yang Min has never before experienced such enormous pressure – threats from officials, police intimidation, house arrest, surveillance. 'They know no restraint, they're capable of anything,' she says quietly. 'They are now telling people I'm not right in the head.' The woman who previously praised the power of the regime has finally come to understand that the regime is not there to make her life easy. On the contrary, it is far more powerful than her suffering.

'Now I am most concerned that I'll implicate my old man if I continue to make a ruckus,' she says. 'He'll surely be dragged into it, right?' She discusses divorce with Mr Tian. 'You go on to live a normal life. I'll get justice for our daughter.' But Old Tian is adamant, telling his wife, 'There's only two of us now. If something happens to you, how will I go on?'

And then there's her other relatives – older brother, older sister – who exhort her to 'live a normal life'.

She is still feeling sorrowful and angry and sometimes thinks, *I'm going to die anyway. Rather than be tormented, I might as well fight to the end.* But when she calms down, she sees the road ahead more clearly. It is a hard road, endless and dangerous. She has no idea if she can make it to the end.

Her determination gradually wavers. On 19 May, she buries Yuxi's ashes in a mountain range not far from Wuhan – something she previously refused to do. She writes on Weibo:

> *You always wanted your own house and now you have one. Daughter, are you happy? I dreamed I saw you find work. You were in such high spirits when you told me. Daughter, are you happy? Your world must be beautiful and blessed. Daughter, are you happy? You will never have to suffer illness again. Daughter, are you happy?*

From the moment Yang Min takes the casket of ashes and walks out of her door, eight men tail her closely. As she arrives at the grave site, the cemetery dispatches several more people. The dozen-odd men resemble an army. They watch Yang Min caress the photograph of her daughter and they watch her collapse to the ground wailing. Perhaps they feel her sadness, but above all else this inconsolably sad mother is their enemy, an enemy of the state.

Since that day, Yang Min rarely has an opportunity to leave the house freely. The tails – some are disguised, some are not, some are gentle while others are forceful – never leave her side and are always ready to strike. Yang Min speaks in a dispirited voice to her friends on Signal: 'I'm now confined. I can't leave the neighbourhood. I can't even go out the gate ... I can't even go out and reason with them.'

'I'm not safe here, but I have no way out,' she sighs softly. 'My strategy now is ... just to survive.'

Little by little, her anger subsides. Crying bitterly, she once vowed to get justice for her daughter, but in the end, just like other 'emotionally stable' family members of the dead, she swallows her sorrow and anger and lives docilely. A psychic tells her Yuxi's departed spirit is not doing well. Yang Min is so concerned that Yuxi will be bullied in the nether world that she goes to a temple to perform ceremonies to help Yuxi's soul find peace. 'After the ceremonies, my child is a lot calmer, so am I,' she murmurs.

As Wuhan's June heatwaves are making people wilt and flowers bloom, Yang Min is still living under surveillance and house arrest. Across the nation, at malls, supermarkets, train stations and airports, everyone has to scan QR codes to record their health details, movements and modes of transport. Yang Min suspects her mobile phone has been tampered with. 'I can never scan the QR codes,' she says. 'Other people scan just once, but when

I try, it just keeps on spinning, but nothing ever appears on the display.'

Almost inaudibly, she says, 'But even if I could scan, they won't let me out, let alone now that the scans don't work.'

From this point on, she does not answer telephone calls from strangers and does not complain anymore in her Signal group. One of her relatives says Yang Min has no further plans for street protests because she cannot go out onto the streets. She is planning to instigate a lawsuit, 'according to normal procedures'.

There are fewer new posts on her Weibo account, or perhaps they are published and no one sees them. On 27 June, she reposts a commentary with just one word: 'Hate'. Several people repost it, but the number is far less than earlier. Perhaps that is why the fifty centers no longer bother to troll her.

About two months later, on 20 August she posts another message, just a few words: 'Bring my daughter back.'

This time there are no comments. For many people in China, the disaster ended a long time ago. There is no need to remember, and it should not be remembered. Autumn is coming, the state TV station says, and autumn is harvest season.

Afterword

By the time of this book's publication, the novel coronavirus has several variants. Wuhan appears to have almost returned to normal. Some shops have closed and, after a paint job, some have reopened. Children born during the lockdown are now learning their first words and the dead are slowly being forgotten. On the sometimes boisterous, sometimes desolate city streets, the people we got to know in this book occasionally make an appearance. They hurriedly go about their business, though most have not fared too well.

Lin Qingchuan is still struggling in that small community hospital. He remains single and is burdened with misgivings about the future. He often works night shifts and is occasionally dispatched to a newly built isolation facility. Over the past year, similar isolation stations have proliferated. They hold many patients, locals as well as travellers from Japan, Hong Kong and beyond. Hard work is not necessarily well remunerated – his pay packet is meagre and the payroll is often delayed. On the way to work he sighs, 'Spinach is 12 yuan a catty' (A$2.65 for 500 grams).

Jin Feng hardly ever visits Wuhan after she returned to the countryside. She has become taciturn and rarely tells anyone her story. She still cherishes the hope that before she dies, she will be able to get her son a disability certificate.

Li the motorcycle taxi driver still waits at the Hankou Railway Station. Over the past year, he has had fewer and fewer passengers. He often needs to borrow money and sometimes is unsuccessful. He will probably have to relinquish his illegal business soon.

Liu Xiaoxiao is still a substitute teacher in Wuhan. He has had a few romances over the past year, but they have all ended badly. He often gambles online and loses some money, but then wins it all back. He says of himself, 'I'm no saint.' His friend Xia Lunwen returned home but hasn't found a stable job. However, Xia did not stop writing poetry. In late 2021, he drifted to China's southernmost island, Hainan, to write a series of epic poems praising the Communist Party and Xi Jinping, as well as those miraculous herbal medicines. In one poem, he wrote that cow dung can treat hernias.

Li Xuewen has been depressed for the past year, though he has managed to write many articles. He appealed for

Zhang Zhan and protested on behalf of his political prisoner friends. Most of his articles are censored. At the end of 2021, he wrote a film script which he hopes to sell to a discerning producer. He says he believes 'the world will not let down people who work hard'.

For Wang Gangcheng and Shao Shengqiang, life continues much as before. They have few worries, but even if they did, they would not talk about them publicly.

Yang Min posts rarely on Weibo and has little contact with the outside world. No one seems to know anything about her current circumstances.

Zhang Zhan now weighs less than 40 kilograms. She has persisted with her hunger strike and is unlikely to end it. In late 2021, her brother posted a heartbroken message on Twitter, writing that Zhang Zhan 'will possibly not live much longer'. He attached a photo of her on a riverbank, smiling. She looks young and full of vitality. 'If she doesn't survive,' her brother wrote, 'I hope the world will remember what she once looked like.'

London,
January 2022

Editor's note

Clive Hamilton

From the earliest days of the emergence of a strange new virus in Wuhan, and for the next five months, I kept a contemporaneous diary of events drawing on Western media, Chinese media and government websites, expert comment and scientific journals. Below is an edited version that provides a helpful background to the first-hand accounts that make up this book. A longer version, with links to sources, can be read at tinyurl.com/4mua48yk.

On 18 November 2019, the Wuhan Institute of Virology posts a notice inviting applications for post-doctoral fellows to join a team experimenting with bats to research Ebola- and SARS-associated coronaviruses.

On 8 December, the Wuhan Health Authority says it has become aware of the first case of a pneumonia of unknown cause. It does not pass on the information. The onset of symptoms of this first patient was 1 December. On 12 December, the Wuhan Municipal Health Commission identifies the first cases of a new coronavirus infection. The commission makes no information public – including to doctors – while it decides what to do and waits for direction.

By 15 December, Wuhan authorities have now recorded twenty-seven cases of patients with the SARS-like illness.

The next day, a sixty-five-year-old patient is transferred from Nanjing Road Hospital to the emergency department of Wuhan Central Hospital with infection in both lungs. It's soon learned that he worked at Wuhan's Huanan (South China) Seafood Market. By 22 December the patient fails to respond to treatment and is transferred to the respiratory department. Two days later, a sample is sent to various labs for analysis.

The Wuhan Institute of Virology posts a second job ad recruiting post-docs to work on the aetiology and transmission of coronaviruses found in bats and rodents, including a project funded by the US National Institutes of Health.

On 25 December, a report in *China Youth Daily* (the official newspaper of the Communist Youth League) claims doctors in two Wuhan hospitals have been isolated after suspected infection with a virus of unknown cause. It's believed they caught it from patients, the first signs of human-to-human transmission. As they worked in respiratory departments, where protections against infection are very thorough, it's thought the virus 'may be very contagious'.

On 26 December, a technician at a lab analysing samples from Wuhan hospitals says his company is shocked to discover a new strain of coronavirus similar to SARS. The next day, Vision Medicals, a genomics company in Guangzhou, phones a doctor at Wuhan Central Hospital to say it has identified a new coronavirus. Records show more than 180 people have now been infected. Wuhan Central Hospital launches an immediate and confidential investigation.

On 30 December, the director of the emergency department at Wuhan Central Hospital, Dr Ai Fen, receives a lab report from another gene sequencing company, CapitalBio Medlab, on a sample taken from a different patient. This patient had no contact with the seafood market. The report includes the words 'SARS coronavirus'. Ai Fen later says she broke into a 'cold sweat'. Circling the words with a red pen, Ai Fen photographs the page of the report and posts it on a WeChat group of medical colleagues. She warns fellow doctors not to visit the seafood market. She also sends it to doctors in her department, urging them to take precautions against a new form of coronavirus.

Within hours the report is circulating among Wuhan doctors. Dr Li Wenliang, an ophthalmologist at Wuhan Central Hospital, reposts Ai Fen's photo of the report to his medical classmates. He asks his colleagues to keep it confidential, but a screenshot of his message soon goes viral.

Dr Ai Fen notifies the hospital's public health department of the lab report. The Wuhan Municipal Health Commission notifies hospitals of a 'pneumonia of unclear cause' and orders them to report any cases. At 10.20 pm Ai Fen receives a message from the hospital informing her that the outbreak is now in the hands of the health commission and ordering that no information is to be released in order 'to avoid causing panic among the people'.

Later that night, at 1.30 am on 31 December, Dr Li Wenliang is summoned to a meeting at the Wuhan Municipal Health Commission. He is interrogated about the 'mistake of spreading rumours' and ordered to write a self-criticism.

The health commission issues a public statement noting that 'Cases of a pneumonia of unknown cause have intermittently surfaced at Wuhan's South China Seafood Market'. The notice says that there is no 'obvious sign of human-to-human transmission' and no medical staff have been infected. Wuhan residents are relieved by the reassurances and carry on as normal.

The commission says twenty-seven cases have been identified. Other confidential government documents indicate the number of confirmed cases has reached 266.

Reporters find the seafood market open and busy. The market is a kilometre from the Hankou Railway Station, a hub for fast trains to Beijing, Shanghai and Hong Kong. Throughout December, tens of thousands of people are also travelling overseas from Wuhan.

In Taipei, the deputy director of Taiwan's Centre for Disease Control notices online chatter among Wuhan doctors and notifies his colleagues. Taiwan begins screening flights from Wuhan and attempts to warn the World Health Organization (WHO) that the new coronavirus is capable of human-to-human transmission.

On 31 December, Wuhan city authorities notify the China office of the WHO that cases of a pneumonia of unknown cause have been detected in Wuhan. A team of experts from the National Health Commission in Beijing arrives in Wuhan.

China's social media censors begin blocking hundreds of words and phrases linked to the outbreak, including 'Wuhan seafood market' and 'SARS variation'.

On 1 January 2020, the South China Seafood Market is shut down in order, authorities say, 'to bring its practices in line with regulation'. Shop owners are forced to leave without emptying their refrigerators.

Dr Ai Fen is summoned to the hospital's supervision department and given a dressing down for 'spreading rumours'. She's instructed to say nothing about the virus, either to her colleagues or even her husband. 'If I'd known what was to happen,' she later revealed in a magazine interview, 'I would not have cared about the reprimand. I would have fucking talked about it to whoever, wherever I could.' (The citizens of Wuhan are known in China for using colourful language.)

Eight doctors, including Li Wenliang, are taken in for questioning by the Wuhan Public Security Bureau. The bureau issues a statement saying the eight 'were investigated and dealt with according to law'. The message has an immediate chilling effect.

WHO requests further information about the influenza of unknown cause.

The Hubei Provincial Health Commission contacts labs testing for the novel coronavirus ordering them to destroy samples and to cease testing. Researchers at the Wuhan Institute of Virology have now sequenced the entire genome of the pathogen, confirming that it is a novel coronavirus. It is three days before they are authorised to provide the information to the WHO.

The next day, China's top health authority, the National Health Commission, orders institutions including the Wuhan Institute of Virology to stop publishing anything about the new virus and to destroy all samples.

Summoned to the police station, Dr Li Wenliang is forced to sign a reprimand and a 'letter of warning' in which he 'repents' illegally publishing untruthful information and promises to cooperate.

On 3 January, China's authorities notify the WHO that forty-four patients with pneumonia of unknown cause have been reported, with eleven severely ill.

Taiwan's health authorities tell doctors to be on the lookout and Singapore begins checking temperatures of travellers arriving from Wuhan. The president of the University of Hong Kong's Centre for Infection indicates it's highly probable the new virus can be spread from human to human, and urges the implementation of a strict monitoring system.

On 5 January, a lab in Shanghai asked to sequence the virus genome is 'shocked' to find a new virus similar to SARS and 'strongly recommended precautions in public places and anti-viral treatment'.

WHO issues a statement saying it is monitoring the situation and advises against imposing any restrictions on travel to and from China. The US Centers for Disease Control and Prevention offers to send experts to China to help identify the disease and its spread. Beijing declines and rejects later offers.

At a meeting of the Politburo Standing Committee on 7 January, General Secretary Xi Jinping issues orders to contain the virus but also decides to suppress knowledge of it. As the virus spreads in the lead-up to the Lunar New Year (Spring Festival), the leaders are opposed to any contingency measures 'that may mar the festive vibe and make the public panic'. Propaganda officials instruct Chinese media to 'prevent false reports from causing panic, do not write conjecture, do not quote foreign news media, do not link to SARS'.

On 9 January, Chinese health authorities and the WHO announce that a novel coronavirus, to be known as 2019-nCoV, is responsible for the Wuhan outbreak and that its genome has been sequenced. In a coordinated move, a number of Twitter and Instagram accounts operated by Chinese state media outlets begin mentioning the Wuhan outbreak for the first time. They emphasise China's transparency and the limited spread of the virus. Tweets from the Party's *Global Times* refer to the virus 'originating in Wuhan'.

On 10 January, *The New York Times* reports that 'no new cases have been detected' since 3 January and 'there is no evidence that it can spread among humans'.

From 5 to 17 January, Chinese authorities do not register any new cases of novel coronavirus, despite hundreds of patients arriving at hospitals in Wuhan and elsewhere in China. Respiratory wards are full and short of protective equipment. Patients have spilled into other wards ill-prepared to treat them.

On 11 January, the Wuhan Health Authority announces the first death from an 'unexplained viral pneumonia', a sixty-one-year-old man who often shopped at the South China Seafood Market. It says forty-one people have been infected with no new cases found after 2 January. Leading a second expert team, Wang Guangfa, director of the respiratory and acute medical department at Peking University First Hospital, reassures Wuhan's citizens that the outbreak is 'preventable and controllable'. Wang himself will soon fall ill with the virus.

A team at Fudan University publishes the genetic sequence of the new pathogen on public databases, the first to do so. A day later, the laboratory is ordered to shut down for 'rectification'.

The National Health Commission passes on the information about the virus's genome to the WHO in Geneva on 12 January. WHO announces that the outbreak is linked to a single seafood market and that no health workers have been infected. It says there is 'no clear evidence of human-to-human contagion'.

Taiwan sends a technical team to Wuhan to investigate, but authorities limit what they can see.

On 14 January, the first overseas case of novel coronavirus is reported in Thailand. China's political leaders begin to take the virus seriously. In Beijing, the Chinese Centre for Disease Control and Prevention

(CDC) begins a national search for cases and orders temperature checks in Hubei's transport hubs and reduction of large public gatherings. But the public is not informed about the severity and transmissibility of the virus.

A top virologist at the Wuhan Institute of Virology, Shi Zhengli, known as 'bat woman' for her work on bat viruses, has found that the new virus can be passed between people, but her information is suppressed. WHO senior coronavirus expert Dr Maria Van Kerkhove says that 'it is very clear right now that we have no sustained human-to-human transmission'. (Three months later she will admit that she suspected human-to-human transmission 'right from the start'.) The Taiwanese technical team leaves Wuhan convinced that 'there is already person-to-person transmission'. WHO tweets that investigations by Chinese authorities 'have found no clear evidence of human-to-human transmission'.

On 15 January, the CDC in Beijing initiates a level-one emergency response. Beijing sends out instructions to embassies and consulates all over the world to mobilise diaspora populations, including overseas Chinese organisations, to buy up as much protective equipment as possible. Over the next several weeks they scour warehouses and retail pharmacies, sending back 2.4 billion items of protective equipment, including two billion masks.

In mid-January, the Chinese military's top epidemiologist and virologist arrives in Wuhan with a team of military scientists. They base themselves at the Wuhan Institute of Virology. While China claims there are now only 300 patients, an analysis by experts at Imperial College London reports that their best estimate of the number of cases of the novel coronavirus is 1700, suggesting substantial human-to-human transmission.

On 18 January, Wuhan Union Hospital calls an emergency meeting to instruct staff to adopt stringent isolation.

Thousands of families gather in Wuhan's Baibuting neighbourhood for the municipality's '10,000-family feast'. Mayor Zhou Xianwang defends the much-criticised decision on the grounds that 'the spread of the epidemic had only limited transmission between people'.

Another team of senior experts sent by the National Health Commission in Beijing has arrived in Wuhan. It's headed by virologist Professor Zhong Nanshan, regarded as a national hero for his work on the 2003 SARS virus. Interviewed on state broadcaster CCTV news on the evening of 20 January, Zhong Nanshan finally confirms that the novel coronavirus can be transmitted between people and that fourteen healthcare workers had caught the virus while treating a single patient. The effect is immediate. Wuhan citizens are furious at being kept in the dark.

General Secretary Xi Jinping instructs State Council to take high-level control and prevention measures.

The 21 January issue of the *People's Daily*, which for weeks has been ignoring events in Wuhan, finally broaches the epidemic and General Secretary Xi's instructions to 'put the people's health and safety first'. A top Party body warns that those responsible for covering up the outbreak would be 'nailed to the pillar of shame for eternity'.

President Xi is reported to have spoken with WHO Director-General Tedros Adhanom Ghebreyesus in Beijing. Western intelligence agencies will later claim that Xi pressured Tedros to delay declaring a public health emergency, threatening to deny cooperation. WHO reports that 278 cases have been identified in China. Confirmed cases have by now been identified in Japan, Thailand, Taiwan, South Korea and the United States.

Early on 22 January, Wuhan officials implement a second-degree public health emergency response. Citizens are required to wear masks in public. There are chaotic scenes at Wuhan No. 5 Hospital, overwhelmed with patients. Many medical workers move into hotels to avoid infecting their families.

Imperial College London advises the WHO that 'human-to-human transmission of the novel coronavirus COVID-19 (previously termed 2019-nCoV) is the only plausible explanation of the scale of the outbreak in Wuhan'.

The next day, US President Donald Trump tweets: 'China has been working very hard to contain the Coronavirus. The United States greatly appreciates their efforts and transparency. It will all work out well. In particular, on behalf of the American People, I want to thank President Xi!'

At 2 am on 23 January, the Wuhan government orders a lockdown of the city. Some rush to the stations and airports to catch the last trains and planes out of the city. The mayor will admit three days later that five million people had already left the city, some to escape the epidemic. A Wuhan doctor says the virus is spreading at an alarming rate and 'hospitals have been flooding with patients, there are thousands'. A radiologist confides to a *Caixin* journalist that 143 out of his 200 colleagues have been infected, along with his wife.

Expressing confidence in China's handling of the epidemic, the WHO says it won't declare a 'Public Health Emergency of International Concern'. Director-General Tedros is the final decision-maker.

Over 40,000 doctors and nurses have arrived in Wuhan from all over China. Hundreds of workers are mobilised to build a makeshift hospital on Wuhan's outskirts, to be ready in six days and able to accommodate one thousand patients. Ma Guoqiang, Wuhan's Communist Party secretary and most powerful official, tells state media that he should have ordered preventive measures earlier. 'I'm in a state of guilt, shame and self-reproach,' he said. Beijing is happy for local officials to take the blame.

Prestigious journal *The Lancet* publishes a study by Chinese scientists indicating human transmission and throwing doubt on the claim that the virus originated in the South China Seafood Market.

Whistleblower Dr Li Wenliang, who has caught the virus, gives an interview to the *Beijing Youth Daily* from his sick bed on 24 January.

On Lunar New Year, 25 January, videos circulate of traumatised hospital doctors collapsing and weeping. Social media platform WeChat announces that it is deploying 'professional third-party rumour removal agencies to refute [coronavirus] rumours'.

On 26 January, Premier Li Keqiang arrives in Wuhan to 'inspect and give guidance' to local officials and hospital workers and to oversee construction of new hospitals. State media announces that the Politburo Standing Committee has formed a top-level group to manage the crisis, to be led by Premier Li Keqiang. It includes Wang Huning, 'Xi Jinping's propaganda chief', and Huang Kunming, head of the CCP's propaganda department.

Popular Wuhan writer Fang Fang reports that masks are in short supply and have replaced pork as the most sought-after New Year gift. Netizens criticise Xi Jinping as 'gutless' for his no show in Wuhan and suggest 'the buns are mentally handicapped', referencing Xi's banned nickname 'steamed bun'. Censors delete the posts. Across China, activists and lawyers are visited by police threatening them with prison if they post about the virus.

On 28 January, hospitals in Wuhan are overflowing with patients, with beds lining corridors and patients dying in waiting areas. Beleaguered medical staff issue desperate calls for help and supplies.

WHO Director-General Tedros meets Xi Jinping in the Great Hall of the People. Tedros is reported expressing his admiration for the Chinese government's political resolve, transparency and timely and effective action.

On 29 January, Wang Liming, a professor at Zhejiang University, takes to Weibo to point out that the CDC in Beijing 'had clear evidence of human-to-human transmission as early as the first days of January'. At what point was this information covered up, he asks. His post immediately goes viral.

Relatives of a patient who'd died at Wuhan No. 4 Hospital attack a doctor, ripping off his mask and shouting, 'If we're sick, we'll be sick together. If we have to die, we'll die together.' It's reported that a seventeen-year-old boy with cerebral palsy has died from hunger and cold after his sole-carer father was taken away and put under quarantine. Distressed by the story, Fang Fang writes that the 'social disease' of officialdom is 'more severe and persistent than coronavirus'.

China's National Health Commission begins excluding from its data patients who test positive for coronavirus but have no symptoms.

Hubei citizen journalist Gao Fei, who had been reporting first-hand about the epidemic, goes missing. He sends out a last video message as police chase him and try to enter his apartment.

By 30 January, the virus has spread to eighteen countries. WHO Director-General Tedros is forced to declare a global public health emergency but advises nations not to restrict travel to or trade with China.

Italy announces its first confirmed cases of the coronavirus, two Chinese tourists who arrived a week earlier. Air traffic with China is suspended. A few days later Italy's ambassador in Beijing is given a dressing down by Vice Foreign Minister Qin Gang for 'overreaction'.

On the last day of January, the WHO's representative in Beijing, Gauden Galea, holds a video briefing for diplomats. After praising China's response, he calls on other countries 'not to step out of line with the WHO recommendations'. He warns that any nation that takes measures beyond those recommended by the WHO 'will have to scientifically justify' them and 'this justification will be made public'.

The United States imposes a limited travel ban for non-citizens arriving from China; Beijing expresses annoyance. On 1 February Australia announces it will refuse all arrivals from China except for Australian citizens, who will be required to enter a two-week quarantine period; the ban is criticised by the Chinese embassy for being imposed too quickly.

Posts circulate on Weibo and WeChat suggesting a researcher at the Wuhan Institute of Virology was the first to be infected by the novel coronavirus. Virologist Shi Zhengli reacts furiously.

From his hospital bed, Dr Li Wenliang tells *Caixin*: 'A healthy society cannot have just one voice.'

In Wuhan, citizen rage is stoked further when 'senior officials were seen on TV news using high-end N95 respirators while frontline doctors made do with disposable medical masks'. Frontline medics are reported to be wearing adult nappies 'so they don't have to waste time taking their biohazard suits on and off when they go to the loo'.

On 3 February, an article by four Chinese scientists published in *Clinical Infectious Diseases* suggests that the virus was carried by wild mammals infected by bats and sold at the Wuhan seafood market.

Xi Jinping gives a speech to a meeting of the Politburo Standing Committee describing his own leading role in fighting the epidemic and praising the Central Committee for getting everything right. He went on to emphasise the need to do 'propaganda and ... public opinion guidance well'.

Forty-two nations have imposed some kind of trade or travel restrictions, and in China authorities are locking down more cities and provinces to prevent the spread of the virus.

In Geneva, WHO Director-General Tedros says: 'There is no reason for measures that unnecessarily interfere with international travel and trade.' He heaps praise on the Chinese government.

A withering criticism of General Secretary Xi's and the Party's response to the epidemic is published by Xu Zhangrun, professor of law at Tsinghua University in Beijing: 'The cause of all of this lies, ultimately, with the Axle Rod [Xi Jinping] and the cabal that surrounds him ... [B]ureaucrats throughout the system consciously shrugged off responsibility for the unfolding crisis while continuing to seek the approbation of their superiors.' Xu is soon silenced.

On 5 February, respected news magazine *China News Weekly* publishes a long article by four investigative journalists exposing the cover-up of the virus over the seven weeks from 1 December to 20 January. Within a day the article has disappeared.

A pre-print of a short paper by two scientists from Wuhan concludes that 'the killer coronavirus probably originated from a laboratory in Wuhan'.

The death of whistleblower Dr Li Wenliang leaks out on Weibo, sparking an unprecedented wave of anger, sadness and grief. Analysts suggest this 'likely marks a turning point in the disillusionment of a generation which previously seemed to accept, without question, the trade-off between openness and stability'. Beijing's censors issue instructions to Chinese media on how to report Li's death.

Chen Qiushi, a lawyer and citizen journalist whose video posts of overwhelmed hospitals and distressed locals attracted millions of views, disappears.

On 8 February, newspapers in China begin rewriting the Li Wenliang case, leaving out his interrogation and humiliation by the police. A popular hero is being moulded into a Party hero.

On Sunday 9 February, Fang Bin, a businessman turned citizen journalist reporting from the heart of the epidemic, disappears.

The next day, the WHO announces that henceforth the official name of the disease will be COVID-19, and SARS-CoV-2 for the virus that causes it. Director-General Tedros says that COVID-19 has been chosen to avoid stigmatising any group and to be pronounceable.

On 13 February, the number of reported confirmed cases in Hubei increases sharply, up by 14,000 to over 60,000, due to a change in how the number of cases is measured. Authorities admit that 1716 medical workers have caught the virus, with at least six doctors dying.

Xinhua reports that Wuhan Party Secretary Ma Guoqiang has been ousted and replaced by Wang Zhonglin. Hubei province Party Secretary Jiang Chaoliang is also replaced.

A pre-print of an article released by scientists in Guangzhou and Wuhan concludes that it's unlikely the virus got into humans from the seafood market: 'In summary, somebody was entangled with the evolution of 2019-nCoV coronavirus. In addition to origins of natural recombination and intermediate host, the killer coronavirus probably originated from a laboratory in Wuhan.' The article is quickly removed.

Xi announces the fast-tracking of a new law for 'biosecurity at laboratories' specifically targeting the use of biological agents that 'may harm national security'. The next day, the Chinese Ministry of Science and Technology publishes a new directive strengthening biosecurity in labs that 'handle advanced viruses like the novel coronavirus'.

A thorough study by twenty-seven Chinese scientists is published in *The Lancet* re-examining forty-one cases admitted to hospital in the early stages of the outbreak, confirming that fourteen of them – including the first person diagnosed with SARS-CoV-2 on 1 December – had no contact with the seafood market and lived a long way from it. Messages have been circulating on WeChat and Weibo claiming that 'patient zero', Huang Yan Ling, was a researcher at the Wuhan Institute of Virology. The institute releases a statement saying that Huang Yan Ling left Wuhan in 2015 and was quite healthy. Her photo and bio have been scrubbed from the institute's website.

A statement from the Ministry of Public Security reports that police have handled 5111 cases of 'fabricating and deliberately disseminating false and harmful information' about the epidemic.

After twelve days being toured around other parts of China, select members of a WHO–China joint mission finally arrive in Wuhan on 22 February. The mission's report has already been drafted. They spend one day in Wuhan where they are chaperoned through two hospitals. In the report (released on 28 February), the WHO team praises General Secretary Xi Jinping and concludes that 'China has rolled out perhaps the most ambitious, agile and aggressive disease containment effort in history'.

On 23 February, Beijing announces a permanent ban on wildlife consumption and trade, other than for research or medicinal purposes.

On 26 February, Communist Party organs publish the first history of the coronavirus crisis, a book titled *A Battle Against Epidemic: China combatting* COVID-19 *in 2020*. It extols Xi Jinping's 'sense of mission, his far-reaching strategic vision and outstanding leadership'.

Virologist Zhong Nanshan, described as China's leading expert on COVID-19 and a party favourite, tells a news conference that while the first infections were reported in China, the virus may not have originated in China.

On 28 February, China Media Project reports that citizen journalist Li Zehua, who had previously worked for CCTV, appears to have been taken into custody by state security after a four-hour stand-off outside his apartment door.

In the first days of March, Beijing sends instructions to its embassies to use Twitter and foreign media to put doubt in people's minds about the origin of the coronavirus, suggesting the message: 'If the coronavirus has been successfully deployed from Wuhan, its real origin remains unknown. We are looking for where it comes from exactly.'

On 3 March, a study by experts at the University of Southampton concludes that if travel bans, social distancing and isolation of infected people had been implemented in Wuhan one week earlier, then the number of cases would have been two-thirds lower.

On 5 March, new Wuhan Party Secretary Wang Zhonglin is embarrassed when, on a visit to Wuhan, Vice Premier Sun Chunlan is heckled by residents who yell from their windows 'fake, fake, everything is fake' as local officials show her around a quarantined neighbourhood. Wang Zhonglin tells officials the people of Wuhan need to be given 'gratitude education' so they can properly express their appreciation to the Communist Party and Xi Jinping for their management of the epidemic. His call sparks a storm of online criticism and backfires badly. On 7 March, a report to an internal CCP propaganda meeting refers to the 'gratitude education' incident, saying it prompted 'raging public opinion' comparable to the uproar that followed the death of Dr Li Wenliang. Party media are told to delete all reference to it, and the newspaper that first carried Wang's remarks, *Changjiang Daily*, is reprimanded.

On 7 March, Fox News anchor Tucker Carlson meets privately with Donald Trump at Mar-a-Lago. The conversation seems finally to 'puncture Trump's bubble' of denial about the seriousness of the situation.

On 9 March, a new study estimates that in the two weeks prior to Wuhan's lockdown on 23 January, 834 air travellers carrying the SARS-CoV-2 virus flew out of the city to airports all over the world.

Xi Jinping visits Wuhan on 10 March for the first time since the epidemic broke out. A local frontline doctor claims that some symptomatic patients were abruptly released from quarantine in order to cut the apparent numbers of sick people for Xi's visit.

After weeks of mounting pressure, and with more than 118,000 cases in 114 countries, WHO Director-General Tedros declares the coronavirus outbreak to be a pandemic, saying WHO had not wanted to 'cause unreasonable fear'.

In Italy, deaths from the virus double in 48 hours to 2158 and the whole country is locked down. On 12 March, a China Eastern Airbus A-350, packed with 30 tonnes of medical supplies and nine Chinese medical specialists, lands in Rome from Shanghai. An army of Twitter bots promoting the hashtags #forzaCinaeItalia (let's go China and Italy) and #grazieCina (thank you China) reaches peak activity. The bots share a video story claiming that Italians are coming onto their balconies to sing the Chinese national anthem; the video will be shown a week later to have been faked.

'Firebrand' Chinese foreign ministry spokesperson Zhao Lijian tells his near 600,000 followers on Twitter that 'It might be US army who brought the epidemic to Wuhan'.

On 17 March, *Nature Medicine* publishes a paper reaching a definite conclusion: 'Our analyses clearly show that SARS-CoV-2 is not a laboratory construct or a purposefully manipulated virus.' Other experts soon say it is not possible on the evidence to reach that conclusion.

On 18 March, after Beijing had been spreading rumours that the origin of the virus may have been in the United States, the prominent Hong Kong microbiologist Yuen Kwok-yung publishes an article saying it's accurate to refer to it as the 'Wuhan coronavirus'. Late in the day, he retracts the article, telling one news outlet: 'Maybe no one loves the country more than I do.' Beijing expels thirteen journalists working for the *New York Times*, *Washington Post* and *Wall Street Journal*, among the foreign journalists with the best sources and deepest insights into China.

Trailing other countries by weeks, Canada finally closes its borders. Health Minister Patty Hajdu had said that based on WHO advice 'there isn't evidence' for the effectiveness of travel bans. Asked whether WHO data could be trusted, she accuses the journalist of 'feeding into conspiracy theories'.

It's reported on 19 March that China's National Supervisory Commission has accused the Wuhan Public Security Bureau of behaving improperly in its treatment of Li Wenliang. The Party's top disciplinary body says that the policemen who arrested Dr Li have been punished and a 'solemn apology' had been sent to Li's family.

In Bergamo, one of the hardest-hit towns in the Italian province of Lombardy where almost two thousand have died from COVID-19, a funeral director says: 'A generation has died in just over two weeks. We've never seen anything like this and it just makes you cry.' A respected Italian professor of pharmacology comments in an interview that GPs in Lombardy had noticed 'a very strange pneumonia … in December and even November … before we were aware of this outbreak occurring in China'. Beijing suggests to diplomats in Europe they begin referring to 'the Italian virus'. In Spanish hospitals, doctors and nurses are so desperate for protective equipment that they are taping plastic garbage bags over their arms and feet. On 21 March, to much fanfare in CCP media, a 'New Silk Road' train carrying 110,000 masks and 766 protective suits departs Yiwu station in Zhejiang province bound for Spain.

Writing in a Philippines newspaper on 22 March, an international law expert argues: 'Under the law on state responsibility, China's suppression of crucial information about COVID-19 is a violation of its international obligations under the 2005 International Health Regulations (IHR), a treaty established under the auspices of the WHO.'

It's reported that China has excluded around 43,000 asymptomatic infected people from its official tally of cases, even though they had been sent into quarantine.

On 23 March, the European Union's top foreign

affairs spokesman, Josep Borrell, writes: 'There is a global battle of narratives going on.' Germany moves to protect struggling companies from unwanted takeovers from China. It's reported on 25 March that Huawei is donating two million masks in Europe, mainly to countries considering whether to permit its equipment to be used in their 5G networks.

On 26 March, long queues form outside Wuhan funeral parlours as grieving families are permitted to collect the ashes of loved ones. Their numbers, along with photos of boxes of urns bought by funeral parlours for ashes, indicate that Wuhan authorities have grossly understated the number of deaths.

On 27 March, President Trump phones President Xi and tweets: 'China has been through much & has developed a strong understanding of the Virus. We are working closely together. Much respect!'

On 28 March, WHO Assistant Director-General Bruce Aylward is interviewed by Hong Kong broadcaster RTHK. When asked if the WHO would consider allowing Taiwan to join the organisation, Aylward pretends not to hear the question then cuts the video link. The video goes viral.

After angrily criticising other nations for closing their borders and 'isolating China', Beijing bans entry of all foreign travellers. In Europe, headlines concerning Beijing's demands for gratitude are souring attitudes to China and shoddy protection equipment sent from China are undermining Beijing's mask diplomacy.

Dr Ai Fen, the emergency department director who warned her colleagues about a SARS-like flu at Wuhan Central Hospital and was reprimanded, is reported on 29 March to have disappeared.

On 31 March, Taiwan appeals to be permitted to join the WHO, arguing that the WHO is obstructing the world from learning from Taiwan's remarkable success in controlling the virus.

In early April, widespread anger builds in India over China's cover up and attempt to present itself as the saviour of the world. On 5 April, London's *Telegraph* reports an investigation revealing that Facebook and Instagram have been flooded with ads of undisclosed origin praising China and attacking the United States.

Ren Zhiqiang, a former Party loyalist and property tycoon, shares among friends (and soon the world) a blistering rebuke of Xi Jinping, denouncing the Party for cheating the WHO and ridiculing its self-flattery and ritualised blindness to the truth, all represented by 'a clown with no clothes on who was still determined to play emperor'. Three days later, Ren Zhiqiang disappears.

UK Prime Minister Boris Johnson is hospitalised with COVID-19. Two days earlier he had joked that 'he was still shaking hands with everyone, including at a hospital treating coronavirus patients'.

Wuhan's South China Seafood Market remains boarded up. An 'unbearable stench' hangs over surrounding streets from the food that's rotted in the refrigerators.

On 7 April the prestigious scientific journal *Nature* apologises for 'erroneously' linking the coronavirus to Wuhan and China. The publisher, Springer-Nature, had previously censored its journals going to China.

In Washington, President Trump lashes out against the WHO's slow reaction to the emergence of the epidemic in Wuhan, hinting that US funding is being reconsidered.

On 8 April, Wuhan ends its eleven-week lockdown. The famously aggressive editor of CCP tabloid the *Global Times* tweets: 'What really messed up the world is failure of the US in containing the pandemic.'

In Beijing, the State Council issues an order for universities to implement strict management of all scientific papers concerning the coronavirus, especially those dealing with its origin. Political vetting is required before publication is permitted.

An online shrine to Dr Li Wenliang, known by some as China's Wailing Wall, has by 13 April accumulated more than 870,000 remembrances and expressions of love and gratitude.

Plans emerge for the publication in English of the widely admired lockdown diary of Wuhan writer Fang Fang, sparking a surge of jingoistic hatred. Hu Xijin, editor of the *Global Times*, wrote that Fang Fang's diary would be used by political forces abroad and that the Chinese people might have to 'pay the price for Fang Fang's fame in the West'. Fang Fang, a Party member, says the vilification has been so intense that it reminds her of the Cultural Revolution.

In a scoop, Josh Rogin of *The Washington Post* reports that in 2018, US embassy officials visited the Wuhan Institute of Virology and sent official warnings about lax security measures in research on coronaviruses, among other viruses.

On 15 April, President Trump announces that the US is suspending its contributions to the WHO, which represents around 15 per cent of the WHO budget (six times more than China's contributions).

On 14 April in Guangzhou, a hub for Africans in China, a McDonald's restaurant apologises for putting up a sign banning black people. It followed the eviction of hundreds of Africans from hotels and apartments after online rumours that they were spreading coronavirus. African ambassadors in Beijing band together to write a letter to China's foreign ministry: 'The singling out of Africans for compulsory testing and quarantine, in our view, has no scientific or logical basis and amounts to racism towards Africans in China.'

By 16 April, global infections exceed two million, with at least 130,000 deaths.

Countries are calling on China to pay for damages arising from the coronavirus. Australian Foreign Minister Marise Payne calls for an independent global review of the origin and early handling of the coronavirus outbreak. Beijing sternly rejects Australia's proposal, saying the idea disrespects 'the Chinese people's tremendous efforts and sacrifices'. It soon begins a series of punitive trade bans.

Wuhan health authorities announce that many COVID-19 deaths in the city had not been counted and the revised figure is 3869, 50 per cent higher than previously announced.

On 20 April, a cluster of cases breaks out in the huge Chaoyang District in Beijing, which includes the CBD.

Republican lawmakers urge the US government to pursue China in the International Court of Justice for violating the 2005 International Health Regulations.

Citizen journalist Li Zehua, who disappeared on 26 February, resurfaces. In a YouTube video he says he had been in enforced quarantine and had been treated well. The *Global Times* escalates its campaign to discredit Wuhan diarist Fang Fang, characterising her as 'a desperate "online celebrity" who lost her dignity as a writer' when she signed a contract with a Western publisher.

The *Global Times* spreads the notion of a US origin and cover-up, seeding the idea that the virus 'was leaked from a US military biochemical laboratory'. It denounces Australia's call for an international inquiry as 'an all-out crusade against China and Chinese culture'.

In Canada, at least one million N95 masks sourced from a Chinese supplier and thousands of swabs used in coronavirus test kits have failed to meet safety standards.

In a strongly worded attack on Western media, on 28 April the *People's Daily* writes: 'Since the outbreak of COVID-19, the World Health Organization (WHO) has repeatedly stressed that the novel coronavirus could have come from just about anywhere in the world.' It says that claims that the coronavirus originated in China are racist and are therefore 'blatant provocations against modern civilization'.

The White House has asked US intelligence agencies to investigate whether China and the WHO concealed evidence about the emergence of the coronavirus. It's also reported that those agencies have 'found no evidence that the Wuhan lab was the cause of the outbreak – only that it is one of a number of scenarios that cannot be ruled out'. US intelligence agencies issue a brief statement on 30 April declaring that 'The Intelligence Community also concurs with the wide scientific consensus that the COVID-19 virus was not manmade or genetically modified'.

Britain's ambassador to the United States expresses support for an inquiry into the origins of the novel coronavirus and the role of the WHO in responding to it. Sweden is reported to be planning to ask the EU to investigate the origin of the novel coronavirus.

In Ottawa, Dr Bruce Aylward, the Canadian physician who led the WHO mission to Wuhan and could not bring himself to acknowledge Taiwan, refuses a request to appear before Parliament's Health Committee.

On the first day of May, Bing Liu, a coronavirus researcher at the University of Pittsburgh School of Medicine, is shot dead in his apartment.

On 3 May, it's reported that two academics in China who expressed support for publication of Fang Fang's *Wuhan Diary* are being investigated by their universities and attacked by online trolls.

By 4 May, COVID-19 deaths worldwide exceed 250,000, including 68,000 in the United States.

A new study of the genetically evolving composition of the virus indicates that it likely first jumped to humans sometime between 6 October and 11 December.

A Change.org petition calling for WHO Director-General Tedros to resign closes with over one million signatures.

It's reported that security police in Hubei are questioning many of the volunteers who helped out during Wuhan's crisis, suspecting them of providing information to foreigners on the number of deaths.

After a cluster of new infections in Wuhan, authorities announce plans to test all eleven million residents within ten days. Experts say it's not possible.

Lawyer turned citizen journalist Zhang Zhan, who has been blogging on events in Wuhan, is arrested on 14 May. She is believed to have been taken to Shanghai's Pudong New District Detention Center and is accused by state security police of 'picking quarrels and stirring up trouble', code for unauthorised reporting.

The translator of Fang Fang's *Wuhan Diary*, Michael Berry, says he has received thousands of angry emails, including death threats.

It's reported on 15 May that WHO Director-General Tedros was encouraged by his advisers at the end of January to use less effusive language praising China's response and Xi Jinping.

In London, an editorial in *The Times* of 16 May calls for the West to confront China and pursue 'conscious decoupling'. Australia's proposal for an international inquiry into the origins and responses to the coronavirus pandemic is gathering international support, with the EU collecting signatures for a motion establishing an inquiry at the meeting of the World Health Authority. The performance of the WHO will also be investigated.

More than 100 million residents of north-east Chinese province Jilin are put into lockdown after outbreaks of COVID-19.

On 19 May, the World Health Assembly adopts without opposition a resolution to establish an inquiry into the origins and responses to the coronavirus pandemic.

COVID-19 cases exceed five million globally, with 340,000 dead.

About the Author

Murong Xuecun (nom de plume of Hao Qun) is one of China's most famous contemporary authors. His work includes *The Missing Ingredient, Leave Me Alone*, and *Dancing Through Red Dust*. He wrote a *New York Times* opinion column from 2011 through 2016 and has also written for *The Guardian*. He lives in Australia.

PUBLISHING IN THE PUBLIC INTEREST

Thank you for reading this book published by The New Press; we hope you enjoyed it. New Press books and authors play a crucial role in sparking conversations about the key political and social issues of our day.

We hope that you will stay in touch with us. Here are a few ways to keep up to date with our books, events, and the issues we cover:

- Sign up at www.thenewpress.com/subscribe to receive updates on New Press authors and issues and to be notified about local events
- www.facebook.com/newpressbooks
- www.twitter.com/thenewpress
- www.instagram.com/thenewpress

Please consider buying New Press books not only for yourself, but also for friends and family and to donate to schools, libraries, community centers, prison libraries, and other organizations involved with the issues our authors write about.

The New Press is a 501(c)(3) nonprofit organization; if you wish to support our work with a tax-deductible gift please visit www.thenewpress.com/donate or use the QR code below.